50p

Collins Gem

P

G000094614

Yvonne Worth

Yvonne Worth has been practising the Pilates technique since 1985, when, as a drama student, she was recommended to her first class at the 'Body Control' studio, in Covent Garden, London. Thrilled to discover an exercise system that was fun, extremely effective and suitable for everyone, she has been working with the technique ever since, encouraging others to do the same!

HarperCollins*Publishers*
Westerhill Road, Bishopbriggs, Glasgow G64 2QT

www.collins.co.uk

First published 2003
This edition published 2004

Reprint 10 9 8 7 6 5 4 3 2 1 0

© The Printer's Devil, Glasgow 2003

ISBN 0-00-718112-4

Images on pp 24 & 25 courtesy of peakpilates.com

Model: Patricia A Ralston

Printed in Italy by Amadeus S.p.A.

Contents

Exercises Lying On Front (Prone)   **116**

INTRODUCTION

What is Pilates?

The Pilates technique is a unique system of body conditioning that stretches and strengthens the muscles, improves flexibility, balance, breathing, posture and alignment. It trains you to recognise your strengths and your weaknesses, while providing you with the means of correcting those weaknesses, thereby strengthening and rebalancing your entire body mechanism. Many other exercise systems work primarily on strengthening the muscles themselves, focussing largely on working the limbs. Pilates, on the other hand, concentrates on strengthening the central core and using the abdominal muscles to control the different movements: it also encourages you to focus your mind as you exercise the body, gradually improving your general awareness, co-ordination and overall alignment.

The Pilates system of exercise, which dates back to the mid-1920s, was an unusual approach to exercise in the West at the time. Drawing its influences from Western and Eastern influences alike, it advocated not only the need for regular physical exercise, but also the necessity of bringing our lives into balance on all levels – insisting that we eat a healthy diet, get plenty of sleep, reduce stress in our lives, and hold a positive attitude in all matters.

Today, the growing interest in maintaining an holistic lifestyle, sustaining a level of health and fitness and achieving a sense of well-being in body, mind and spirit, has led to an ever-increasing popularity in the principles and practice of Pilates.

A further reason for the current popularity of the Pilates system is its potential to change the body shape. Pilates works to stretch and lengthen the muscles, encouraging the body to become stronger

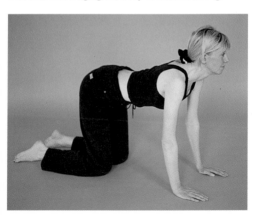

and firmer, but without the disadvantage of also building unwanted bulk. The technique also works to improve posture, thereby allowing you to use your body more effectively and efficiently, even when carrying out mundane daily activities.

Moreover, Pilates does not require you to give up your current fitness routine. Quite the opposite, it was always intended as a system that would work in conjunction with other exercise programmes: strengthening, rebalancing and realigning the body, while also improving body awareness and therefore reducing the risk of strain or injury that can so easily occur in many other forms of exercise. Indeed, Pilates is recommended as a complement to other exercises, not a substitute: even the most dedicated Pilates student is recommended to also incorporate some form of cardiovascular exercise into his or her weekly routine.

Finally, because the exercises are all adaptable to the needs of the individual, a major attraction of Pilates is that it is suitable for anyone, regardless of age, size or level of fitness. It is also enormously beneficial to those who have never previously undertaken any exercise programme, and to those who are wishing to rehabilitate following an injury.

HISTORY OF PILATES

Joseph Hubertus Pilates was born in 1880, near Dusseldorf, Germany. As a child he was extremely frail, suffering from various conditions including rickets, asthma and even rheumatic fever. Determined to overcome his ill health and lead a healthy life, he engaged in a programme of rigorous exercise, exploring various disciplines and activities, including gymnastics, body-building, wrestling, diving and skiing. Taking selected elements from various different activities he devised a programme of fitness that would help him achieve his maximum possible level of fitness, strength and flexibility.

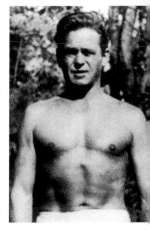

In 1912 Pilates, aged 32, decided to move to the UK, where he earned his living as a boxer, circus performer and a self-defence instructor to detectives. During the First World War he was taken prisoner, due to his German identity. Interned in a camp on the Isle of Man, his duties in the hospital gave him the opportunity to reconsider his fitness routine, adapting the exercises to the various needs of his fellow inmates. Pilates began experimenting with equipment for the first time, constructing simple pieces of equipment from the materials available, e.g. attaching bed springs to the walls so that internees could use the springs to exercise while still lying on their beds.

After the war Joseph Pilates returned to Germany, where he continued to develop his fitness system. Initially he was employed to work with the local police force but eventually he was drafted into the army. In 1926, unable to tolerate the political climate in Germany any longer, he set sail for America. On board ship he met a young woman, Clara, who would later become his wife.

Once in New York, Joseph, with Clara's help, set about establishing his first exercise studio. The location was 939 Eighth Avenue. Very little is known about the studio's early years, but by the 1940s Pilates had achieved great popularity in the performance world with his extraordinary technique – dancers, gymnasts, athletes and actors alike were drawn to his studio. By the 1960s many of New York's top dancers were regular visitors, including George Balanchine, from the New York City Ballet, who proved such an enthusiast of Pilates' approach, that he took the step of inviting him to work with the young ballerinas at the NYC Ballet.

In the past few decades the Pilates technique has continued to grow in popularity, both with professionals (such as performers and sportspeople) for whom fitness is a vital part of their working life and with those members of the general public who have an interest in fitness and well-being. In the past few years, the fascination with the Pilates system has accelerated enormously and nowadays, along with the various dedicated Pilates studios, and individual instructors, many fitness, sports and leisure centres offer classes in the Pilates technique.

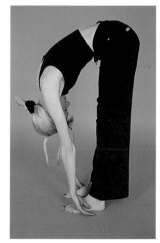

Joseph Pilates' original set of exercises, developed in the 1920s, was made up of 34

moves and manifests influences from eastern and western disciplines alike – the natural result of Pilates' years of studying many different methods of exercise and fitness. However, his routine did not simply consist of a particular set of physical movements to be repeated mindlessly: a fundamental element in the philosophy of Pilates is that true fitness and well-being can only be achieved through an integration of the mind and the body. Pilates himself advocated that, along with an ongoing commitment to regular exercise, each of us should be prepared to examine and alter the various aspects of our daily lives and work towards improving our overall fitness and sense of well-being, both physically and mentally.

The Pilates exercises were never formalised or given an exact form, rather Pilates believed that his moves and routines should be able to be adapted to suit the needs of any individual, whether young or old, large or small, regardless of level of ability or fitness. The result of this has been that Pilates' followers have been able to take the principles of his original teachings and develop their own version of the technique, depending upon their own particular interests and influences. Thus, although the actual manner in which the Pilates method is now taught may vary in both style and emphasis, the fundamental principles of the technique remain unchanging.

PHYSIOLOGY

Skeleton, Bones & Joints

THE SKELETON

The skeleton can be classified into two separate parts:

1. The **axial**, or central, skeleton – this is made up of the head, thorax and vertebral column (spine);

2. The **appendicular** skeleton, or the extremities – this is made up of the bones of the upper and lower body and the pelvis.

THE SPINE

The spine (or vertebral column), skull, ribs and sternum, make up the axial skeleton. The spinal column is comprised of 33 bones, known as vertebrae: seven cervical vertebrae (the neck), 12 thoracic vertebrae (the upper back), five lumbar vertebrae (the lower back), five sacral vertebrae, which are fused together to make one bone called the sacrum (located at the base of the spine), and 4 coccygeal vertebrae, which are fused into one or two bones called the coccyx (the tailbone). The vertebrae are separated

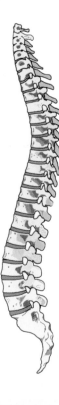

FUNCTIONS OF THE SKELETON:

- to support the body
- to protect the internal organs
- to manufacture red and white blood cells
- to store minerals, particularly calcium and phosphate
- to facilitate movement (which is made possible by the attachment of muscles onto the different bones)

from each other by intervertebral discs, which are made up of fibrocartilaginous material.

The natural shape of the spinal column is actually a slight 'S'. The spine itself both supports the weight of the body and gives the body its basic posture. It also provides protection for the spinal cord and spinal nerve roots. The natural curves of the spine and the intervertebral discs allow the spine to function rather like a spring, making action more agile and absorbing any shock impact to the body. When the spinal curves are altered in any way (for example, repeatedly sitting in an uncomfortable, badly aligned position), stresses are placed on the spine that can lead to bad posture and, eventually, to pain.

The Muscles of the Body

CREATING MOVEMENT WITHIN THE BODY

The central section of any muscle is made up of bundles of thin, parallel fibres, surrounded by a layer of connective tissue. Each muscle fibre has a nerve ending (motor end plate), which receives messages from the brain instructing the muscle to contract. In instances of major muscle movement, such as in the large thigh muscles, one nerve ending will serve numerous muscle fibres, whereas, for fine movements, such as delicate movements of the fingers, a single nerve ending will supply only a few fibres.

Muscle fibres function in a very simple manner – they are either 'switched on' (stimulated) or 'switched off' (not stimulated). Therefore, the degree of muscular contraction is not dependent not upon the extent of the fibre stimulation, but upon the actual number of fibres stimulated – the more fibres that are 'switched on', the greater the degree of contraction.

THE MUSCLE TYPES

The body contains three different muscle types:

- **Cardiac** muscle – found only in the heart.
- **Smooth** (or involuntary) muscle – found in the gut and intestines. These muscles work to process food through the digestive system, and function without our conscious control.
- **Striped/striated** (voluntary) muscle – these muscles are connected to the bones and contract and release to create movement in the body.

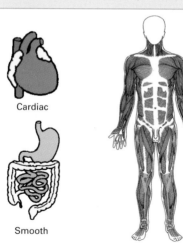

Cardiac

Smooth

Striated

Equally, muscles cannot push, they can only pull, and so the only way they are able to function effectively is by working in opposing pairs. When one pair of muscles contracts, or shortens, the other pair relaxes, or stretches. This system creates the body's ability to move.

THE STRETCH REFLEX

The muscle is provided with a protective mechanism called a stretch reflex. This mechanism is triggered when any muscle is stretched too quickly. Each muscle contains cells that are known as 'muscle spindles'. When a muscle is stretched too fast, and is therefore at risk of tearing, the muscles spindles are activated, automatically triggering the muscle concerned to contract and thereby avoiding injury to the muscle. It is for this reason that, when exercising, it is essential for us to ease into any stretching movement slowly and gradually.

PRINCIPLES OF PILATES

THE FUNDAMENTAL PRINCIPLES OF THE PILATES METHOD

- concentration
- control
- breathing
- flowing movement
- centring
- precision
- awareness

CONCENTRATION

The Pilates technique is not a system of mindlessly repeated exercises in which your body runs on automatic while your mind switches off completely. On the contrary, exercising under the Pilates system requires a great deal of focus and concentration. The mind and body must work together, with the mind remaining alert as each aspect of every movement is carefully controlled and monitored.

CONTROL

In order for us to maintain correct posture and alignment as we work the various different muscles, it is essential for us to acquire good muscle control. In Pilates we exercise to strengthen the body by working against gravity using slow and controlled movements – the slower we are able to work any particular movement, while keeping the move controlled, the stronger the body will gradually become.

BREATHING

Correct execution of the Pilates exercises requires us to use appropriate breathing. Many people have learned to hold their breath as they exercise, or to take shallow breaths into the upper chest, causing a build-up of tension in the body, inhibiting the supply of oxygen to the muscles and reducing the performance of the muscles. In Pilates we breathe deeply, into the lower ribs and the back, moving our muscles in a slow, even rhythm in time with the breathing.

CENTRING

The body's centre, or centre of gravity, is also referred to as the central or abdominal core, or even, sometimes, the powerhouse. The Pilates system considers the body's place of power and control to be here, at the body's centre of gravity (an area approximately 6cm/2in below the navel, also known in some disciplines as the 'hara'). Under the Pilates system, all moves are controlled by the contraction of the muscles located here – the abdominal muscles: if we work from this central core we learn to lengthen and stretch our muscles without risk of strain or injury.

PRECISION

The effectiveness of the Pilates exercises relies on precise execution of each move, and this can only be achieved with a great deal of concentration, patience and practice. As with any new discipline, when you start learning Pilates it can be extremely difficult to remember the various different points, but, with practice, controlling your muscles while keeping your abdominals contracted and your spine in neutral, and stretching and lengthening your muscles in rhythm with your breathing will start to occur automatically.

FLOWING MOVEMENTS

The aim with all the Pilates exercises is to make them as even and flowing as possible, without jarring or jerky movements. Each of the sequences or repetitions of the moves should be controlled throughout by the abdominals and performed using a continuous, slow, smooth, flowing movement, in rhythm with the breathing.

AWARENESS

A keen awareness of the different parts of our physical body is essential if we are to perform the various Pilates moves effectively. Under the Pilates system, it is essential that we develop the ability to listen to our bodies and be guided by what we learn. Exercise is not meant to be a punishment, but a way of improving our fitness and general well-being. An increased awareness will allow us to make sure that we are practising the exercises in a controlled manner, while maintaining correct posture, breathing and alignment, and also working at the appropriate level for our own ability.

PILATES FOR YOU

The Pilates system of exercise can be easily adapted to suit your own particular schedule and preferences. The matwork movements provide you with a thorough programme of exercises, which can be done in the privacy of your own home. This gives you the advantage of adapting your exercise sessions to fit around your other commitments. To have any real effect, Pilates should be practised a minimum of one hour a week, but how you choose to do this is up to you. You may prefer one long session each week, or it may suit you to do shorter sessions more frequently: either two to three 15–20 minute sessions per week, or a daily 5–10 minute session.

COURSES AND CLASSES

You can, of course, successfully workout at home, but, if you find that you would prefer not to exercise on your own, or you simply decide that you would like to work under the guidance of a qualified instructor or expand your knowledge of the Pilates technique, there are many excellent courses and classes available to you. You have the choice of going to a specialist Pilates studio, of which there are many, or attending some of the various classes on offer at a large number of sports, fitness and leisure centres. The majority of Pilates teachers will also give you the option of either group or private sessions.

Learning with an experienced Pilates instructor to guide you is extremely beneficial, as they are fully qualified to assess your particular needs and will be able to guide you and monitor your progress. So, even if your intention is to workout at home, you might consider enrolling on at least a short course of Pilates classes or even taking some one-to-one sessions.

WORKING WITH EQUIPMENT

Joseph Pilates' original routine consisted of a mixture of exercises, some of which would be done on the floor and others that would be performed using his specially designed exercise equipment. Nowadays, many teachers work purely using matwork exercises, with the aid of some very simple pieces of equipment, such as tennis balls and rubber exercise bands, but there is also the option of attending a well-equipped Pilates studio and working with the exercise machinery too. This is rather like visiting a gym, although the equipment is quite different in design and many of the machines use springs, rather than weights, to provide you with added resistance as you exercise. The atmosphere of most Pilates studios is also very

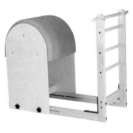

(image courtesy of Peak Pilates™)

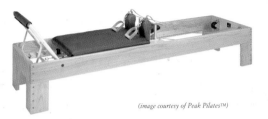

(image courtesy of Peak Pilates™)

different to that of a regular gym, tending to be calm and stress-free, frequently with relaxing music playing in the background. Also, students always work under the strict guidance of a qualified instructor.

BOOKS, VIDEOS AND DVDS

With the rapidly growing popularity of the Pilates technique, there is an ever-increasing number of excellent books, videos and DVDs available today (some of which are listed on pages 184–9). These will give you the opportunity to learn more about Pilates and the different approaches and give you the chance to develop your exercise routine to suit your own needs and preferences. The approach of different instructors can vary, as each may choose to focus on a slightly different system or element of the Pilates method – some even combine Pilates with other disciplines, such as yoga or the Alexander Technique.

PREPARATION

CAUTION

If you suffer from any complaint, are recovering from illness or injury, are pregnant, or have recently lost or gained weight, it is essential that you seek medical advice before committing yourself to any new exercise programme.

Also, if you do suffer from any complaints, if you have never tried a fitness routine before, or if a new exercise programme is part of a major change in your lifestyle, you are advised to consider attending classes where you can work under the instruction of an experienced teacher.

Breathing

Breathing correctly results in an increased efficiency of oxygen supply to the muscles. Many of us have developed the habit of breathing primarily into the chest, raising the ribcage upwards as we inhale. Under the Pilates system, the breathing action is focussed on the lower part of the ribcage and the back. As we breathe in, instead of lifting the ribs upwards, we expand them out to the side and out at the back, breathing deeply to take air to the bottom of the lungs, as far as possible. The chest is not involved in this action and remains as relaxed as possible. This method of breathing is known as 'thoracic' or 'lateral' breathing and, in Pilates, is sometimes referred to as breathing 'full and wide'.

THORACIC BREATHING

1. Stand with your feet in parallel, hip-width apart, your weight centred and evenly distributed over both feet. Place the palms of your hands at the base of your ribs, with the middle fingers of your left and right hands touching slightly. Relax your shoulders and draw your shoulderblades down into your back. Your legs should be straight, but make sure that you are not locking your knees – keep them 'soft' (slightly bent).

2. Breathe in, keeping the chest relaxed and the shoulders down, focus on the lower part of the ribcage. As you inhale, imagine that your ribcage is expanding out to the sides and out at the back. As your ribcage expands, your fingers and hands will separate slightly. Breathe out, relaxing the ribcage and allowing the hands to return to the starting position. Repeat several times, but avoid overdoing it and hyperventilating, particularly if this technique is very new to you.

If you start to feel dizzy, stop immediately

The timing of the breathing is also important in Pilates – whether we breathe in or out as we move can change the quality of the movement itself. The general rule is that we breathe in to prepare, breathe out to move and breathe in to recover.

Co-ordinating the movements of the body with the breathing pattern requires us to establish a rhythm, both in our movement and our breathing. All movements should be smooth and even and performed in perfect time with the breath.

Posture

Correct posture is essential to Pilates. Most of us have learned various bad habits over the years, causing stress to our bodies and resulting in stiffness, tension and even pain. Pilates offers us the means to re-educate our bodies and correct any weaknesses or bad habits. In practising Pilates we focus continually on working with the body in the correct alignment, using the central core to support us as we move. This means that, over time, our posture automatically improves and we begin to find ourselves standing with our spine in good alignment, our shoulders relaxed and our weight evenly spread over both feet. Consequently, no matter what activity we are doing, we will automatically choose a position in which the body can function at its best without risk of strain or injury to any of the muscles or joints.

The Neutral Position

Working from what is known as the neutral position, or neutral spine, is one of the key elements in the Pilates method. This is the term used to describe the position of the body when our spine is in its correct alignment. This is not a precise posture, as each person is different and will therefore have a slightly different natural, or neutral position. However, when correctly aligned, the spine forms a slight 'S'-shape, which is made up of three natural curves – the neck (cervical vertebrae), the upper back (thoracic vertebrae) and the lumbar spine (lumbar vertebrae).

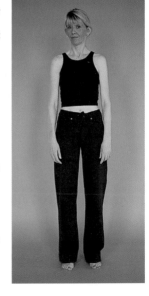

The neutral position

Using the Pilates technique, it is essential to develop the ability to find and maintain this neutral spine position while standing, sitting, or lying down.

STANDING IN THE NEUTRAL POSITION

1. Stand with your feet in parallel, hip-width apart, legs straight and knees soft, shoulders relaxed and down, and arms resting by your sides. Check that your weight is evenly distributed over both feet with your knees positioned directly above your ankles.

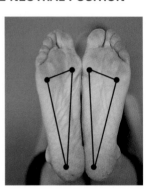

Keep your feet balanced on this triangle on the base of your foot

2. Make sure that your head is balanced correctly on the top of the spine and that you are not jutting your chin forwards or pulling your head back. Draw the shoulderblades down into your back and keep your shoulders relaxed and down away from your ears, without either pulling them back or rounding them forward.

3. Now imagine that there is a thread running through

THE FEET

As we stand, our body should be centred, with our weight evenly distributed over both feet. It is also important that our weight is correctly focused on the feet, and that we are not leaning back and carrying too much weight on our heels, leaning forward and taking too much weight on our toes, or leaning to one side and focusing too much weight on one foot.

- Imagine that there is a triangle on the base of each foot with one side of the triangle running between the big toe and the little toe, and the other two sides running from each of these toes down to the heel. Think of this triangle as your base and concentrate on distributing your weight evenly over this, allowing your body to centre itself correctly over your feet. (See p. 29.)

- Keep the feet flat on the floor – make sure you do not roll them either inwards or outwards.

- Avoid clenching the toes: keep them relaxed and lengthened.

your spine, with one end coming out of the top of your head and travelling up towards the ceiling, and the other coming out through your tailbone down to the floor. Allow this image to help you lengthen all the way along the spine and neck as you imagine sending the crown of your head up to the ceiling and your tailbone down to the floor.

4. You are now standing in what is known as the neutral position. Your back is neither flattened-out nor arched forwards, but correctly aligned, in a slight 'S' shape, following its own natural curves.

5. If you wish, try flattening your back out and then arching it forwards a few times, until you are confident you have found the middle, 'neutral', point.

SITTING IN THE NEUTRAL POSITION

1. Sit on the edge of a chair, with your feet flat on the floor, hip-width apart, your hands either relaxed by your sides or resting on your thighs. Tilt your pelvis forward and round your back, flattening out your lumbar spine and curving the body forward very slightly.

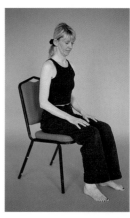

2. Next, tilt your pelvis backward, and arch your lower back.

3. Keep moving between these points until you find the mid position (neutral), with your back straight and a slight natural curve in your lower back.

FINDING THE NEUTRAL POSITION WHILE LYING DOWN

1. Lie on your back with your feet hip-width apart, knees pointing up to the ceiling, your arms by your sides, palms facing down.

2. Tilt your pelvis forward, flattening your lower back, raising your tailbone up away from the floor and lifting your ribs.

3. Now arch your lower back, pressing your tailbone down into the floor and lifting the lower spine away from the floor.

4. Move between these two points until you find your neutral position, with your tailbone on the floor and a slight gap between your waist and the floor – just sufficient for you to slide your hand under your lower back (opposite).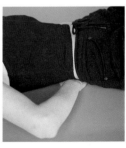

5. Once you have found your neutral position your hips should remain level and stable – as you start to engage in any movement from this neutral position, make sure that you do not twist the pelvis or lift up on one side.

The Abdominal Core

A fundamental factor of the Pilates system is for all exercises to be performed with the support and control of the central, or abdominal core. The aim of Pilates is to create a strong, stable centre from which we can perform our entire range of movements. Focusing on supporting the movement from our abdominal, or central core, allows us to exercise the body while giving support to the lower back, thereby reducing any risk of stress or strain to the lower spine.

To create this core support, before we begin any movement, we first contract the abdominals. Under modern-day Pilates systems, this is achieved by pulling the pelvic floor muscles upwards and inwards (a feeling similar to that of attempting to interrupt the flow of urine) as we draw the abdominal muscles back towards the lumbar spine. Some teachers refer to this as 'navel to spine' or even 'zip and hollow' (i.e. 'zip' up with the pelvic floor muscles and 'hollow' the abdominals back towards the spine). Remember, as you contract the abdominals, be sure to keep your back in the neutral position and avoid rounding out the lumbar spine.

WARMING UP

Warming up is an important element in any exercise routine and should never be missed out. It allows you to gently stretch and mobilise the body, increasing the circulation and activating and warming the muscles in preparation for the more intensive exercises ahead.

Breathing

1. Lie on the floor with your knees bent and pointing straight up to the ceiling, feet flat on the floor in parallel. Place your hands on your lower ribs, elbows pointing out to the sides. Drop your shoulders and draw your shoulderblades down into your back. Make sure that your spine is in neutral and your back and neck lengthened.

2. Breathe in, as deeply as you can, into the lower ribs and the back. You should be able to feel the movement of your ribs under your hands as your ribs expand out to the sides, and the slight pressure of your back against the floor as it expands. Breathe out and release.

4. Repeat 5 to 10 times, trying to increase the movement of the ribs each time. Keep the chest relaxed throughout – do not hunch the shoulders or tense the neck as you breathe.

Rolling Down The Wall

1. Stand with your back against a
   wall or door, feet in parallel,
   hip-width apart, heels
   approximately 12–18 inches
   away from the wall. Drop your
   shoulders and let your arms
   hang relaxed by your sides.

2. Bend your knees slightly,
   tucking your pelvis under and
   take a deep breath. Exhale,
   contract your abdominals, bend
   your head forwards, and slowly
   start to roll down through the
   spine, peeling your spine away
   from the wall vertebra by
   vertebra, directing the top of
   your head straight down
   towards the floor. Keep your knees bent and your
   arms and hands relaxed. If you run out of breath
   pause, take another breath, and continue rolling all
   the way down to the floor, increasing the bend in
   your knees, if necessary.

3. Breathe in, contract the abdominals and start to roll
   slowly back up through the spine, vertebra by
   vertebra, again taking an extra breath if necessary.
   Keep your head bent forwards until the last
   moment. Repeat 5 times.

Standing Balance

1. Stand with your feet slightly apart, knees soft, spine in neutral. Lengthen along the spine and back of the neck. Drop your shoulders, draw your shoulder-blades back and down behind you and relax the arms. Focus your eyes straight ahead and breathe in.

2. Breathe out, contract the abdominals, and continue lengthening up through the spine, allowing your heels to raise up away from the ground. Imagine the top of your head lifting straight up towards the ceiling while at the same time your tailbone releases down to the floor. Remember to keep your eyes directed straight ahead, this will help you balance.

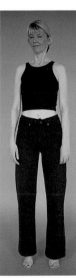

3. Keep rolling up through your feet as you breathe out, until you are balanced on your toes. Do not let your ankles bend out to the sides as you raise up.

4. When you have raised up as far as possible, breathe in, lengthening up through the spine as much as you possibly can.

5. Breathe out, contract the abdominals and slowly lower yourself back down, continuing to lengthen up through the spine as you do so. Repeat 5 to 10 times.

Arm Swings

1. Stand with your feet in parallel, hip-width apart, and your spine in neutral. Lengthen along the spine and neck, breathe in and raise your arms up towards the ceiling, directing them away from the body very slightly. Keep your shoulders dropped and your shoulderblades pulled down into your back.

2. Breathe out, contract the abdominals and swing your arms downwards and then back behind you, bending your knees, relaxing your head and shoulders, bending your head forwards and curving the spine over as you do so.

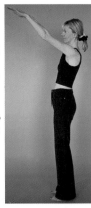

3. Breathe in and slowly swing the arms back and roll back up to the starting position. Repeat the swings 5 to 10 times in a continous, controlled, smooth movement, lengthening the spine up towards the ceiling a little more each time as you roll back up to standing.

Arm Raises Into Arm Circles

1. Stand with your feet in parallel, slightly apart. Place your left hand on your right rib cage to make sure that you do not raise your ribs up as you lift your arm. Breathe in and raise your right arm in front of you, slightly to the side.

2. Breathe in and allow your right arm to raise up, floating your right hand up towards the ceiling. Lengthen the arm out of the shoulder joint as you lift. Keep your shoulder dropped and your ribs soft.

3. Breathe out and slowly lower your arm. Repeat the sequence 5 times.

4. Breathe in and raise your right arm as before, then, as you breathe out, take the arm over and back to the starting position, in a circular motion. Keep your shoulder down, reducing the size of the circles if necessary.

5. Repeat 5 times, keeping the circles slow and even, in time with the breathing, then reverse the direction for 5 more circles.

6. Repeat the sequence for the left arm.

OPTION

Repeat the sequence once more, this time using both arms together. Begin by raising and lowering the arms 5 times and then circle the arms 5 times in each direction, breathing in as you circle the arms up and breathing out as you circle them back down to the starting position. You will find that when circling both arms together you will probably need to make the circles smaller, in order to keep your shoulders dropped throughout the move.

Shoulder Hunches

1. Stand with your feet in parallel, hip-width apart, arms by your sides, spine in neutral.

2. Breathe in to a count of 2 and hunch your shoulders up to your ears, as high as you can. Keep your arms relaxed and your spine and neck in neutral throughout.

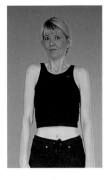

2. Breathe out to a count of 4 as you slowly drop your shoulders back down away from your ears.

3. Repeat the sequence 5 times trying to drop your shoulders a little more each time.

Alternate Hip Openings

1. Lie on your back with your feet in parallel, hip-width apart, your spine in neutral. Place your hands palms down on your abdomen, fingertips on your pubic bone and your thumbs touching, to form a triangle. As you drop each knee out to the side, the area under your hands should stay completely level. Breathe in.

2. Breathe out, contract the abdominals and, keeping your foot in position, slowly let your right knee drop 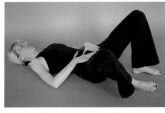 out to the side a little, opening out the hip joint. As you drop the knee, check that your tailbone does not tilt up, and make sure that your hips stay level, with both buttocks in contact with the floor: if your left hip starts to raise up, then you are dropping the right knee too far. Your left leg should remain stable throughout, with your left knee pointing up towards the ceiling.

3. Breathe in as you return the knee back to the starting position. Repeat 5 times on the right side then change legs and repeat 5 times on the left.

Hip Folds

Make sure that you keep your abdominals contracted and your spine in neutral as you 'dip' each foot in turn

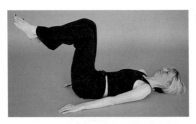

Option 1

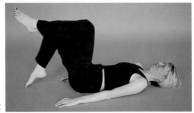

Option 2

1. Lie on your back with your feet in parallel, hip-width apart, knees bent and pointing up to the ceiling, your spine in neutral and your arms by your sides. Breathe in.

2. Breathe out, contract your abdominals and float your right knee up until the knee is at a right angle, with the shin parallel to the floor.

3. Breathe in, holding this position, then breathe out as you lower your foot back down to the floor. Repeat 10 times, alternating the legs each time.

OPTION 1

1. Breathe out as you contract the abdominals and float the right knee up as above. Breathe in, then breathe out and float the left leg up to join it.

2. Breathe out and lower the right foot to the floor, breathe in, then breathe out and lower the left foot.

3. Repeat the sequence, this time raising the left leg first. Repeat the entire sequence 6 to 10 times.

OPTION 2

1. Breathe out as you contract the abdominals and float the right knee up as above. Breathe in, then breathe out and float the left leg up to join it.

2. Breathe out then, using a continuous movement, lower the right foot towards the floor, toes softly pointed, and very gently touch the toes of your right foot onto the floor (as if you were dipping your toes into a pool of water) then raise your leg back up to join the right. Repeat for the left leg.

3. Repeat the toe dips 5 times on each leg, alternating the legs each time.

Egyptian Arm Circles

2

You may place a flat cushion under your head to keep the spine and neck in good alignment

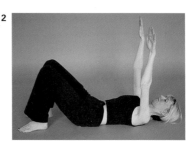

Keep your knees in parallel, pointing straight up to the ceiling as you move the arms

The lower body should stay relaxed throughout

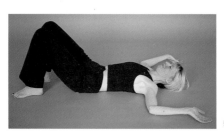

5

1. Lie on your back with your knees bent, feet flat on the floor in parallel, hip-width apart, arms by your sides, palms down. Check your spine is in neutral.

2. Breathe out, contract the abdominals and float your hands up towards the ceiling, until they are level with your shoulders, keeping your arms straight and your elbows soft. Breathe in.

3. Breathe out, bend your elbows so that they are at right angles and bring your upper arms down to the floor, in line with your shoulders, forearms and hands still pointing up towards the ceiling.

4. Breathe in and bring your forearms down to the floor, so that they lie either side of the head, palms facing upwards, elbows at right angles.

5. Breathe out as you continue the movement, straightening your elbows as you lengthen the arms away from you along the ground until they are in parallel, hands shoulder-width apart, then float them up to the ceiling, keeping the elbows straight, until the arms are back in the starting position, with the arms at shoulder level, fingers pointing straight up to the ceiling. Breathe in.

6. Repeat 5 times, then repeat 5 times in the opposite direction, breathing out as you take the arms above the head and down to the floor, breathing in as you bend the elbows, breathing out as you lift the hands and forearms, then straighten the arms, taking your hands straight up towards the ceiling.

STANDING EXERCISES

Rolling Down

Keep your abdominals contracted to focus the strengthening effect of the move and provide support for your lower back

If you have a back problem, seek medical advice before attempting this move

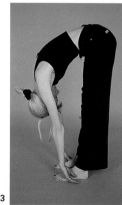

3

BENEFITS

- Strengthens the abdominals and the spine
- Increases flexibility in the back
- Releases tension in the back and shoulders

1. Stand in neutral with your feet hip-width apart, your knees soft (slightly bent) and your weight evenly balanced over both feet. Lengthen through the spine, thinking of sending the crown of your head up to the ceiling and your tailbone down to the floor. Breathe in and contract your lower abdominals.

2. Breathe out, drop your chin onto your chest and start to roll slowly down through the spine, letting the weight of your head draw you down towards the floor. Keep your arms relaxed and your knees soft and avoid sticking the tailbone out – keep thinking of sending it down to the floor.

3. Roll down at a slow, even pace: if you run out of breath, pause and inhale, then exhale and continue rolling the rest of the way down to the floor. Think of curling down through the spine one vertebra at a time, starting at the top and working all the way down to the tailbone.

4. When you have gone as far as you are comfortably able, breathe in, contract the abdominals and breathe out as you reverse the process and slowly roll back up through the spine, to a standing position. Leave your head dropped forwards until the last moment. Again, if you run out of breath, pause and inhale, then exhale and continue to roll back up to standing.

Arm Raises

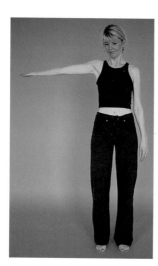

3

Keep the spine lengthened and the body facing forwards

Avoid leaning to one side or swaying backwards or forwards as you lift the arms

Make sure your weight stays evenly balanced over both feet

If you find it difficult to lift the arms to shoulder level while keeping the body in the correct position then take them lower until your strength and muscle control improves

BENEFITS

- Improves posture
- Strengthens the arm and shoulder muscles
- Relieves tension in the neck and shoulders
- Improves breath control

1. Stand with your feet hip-width apart and your spine in neutral, arms relaxed by your sides.

2. Breathe in as you lengthen through the spine and neck, drop the shoulders and draw the shoulder-blades down into your back.

3. Breathe out and slowly raise your right arm out to the side up to shoulder level, lengthening it away from you, keeping the elbow soft and the hand relaxed, palm facing down. Keep the shoulders dropped down, away from your ears, and the shoulderblades drawn back and down behind you as much as possible as you lift.

4. When your arm is at shoulder level, rotate your arm so that the palm faces up to the ceiling.

5. Breathe in as you rotate the hand back and then lower your arm. Repeat 3 to 5 times.

6. Repeat for the other side. Then repeat the sequence once more, raising both arms at the same time.

Waist Twist
(Cossack Arms)

Avoid rounding the shoulders forward, or leaning back as you twist round and release the back

Keep the shoulders dropped and the shoulderblades drawn down into the back

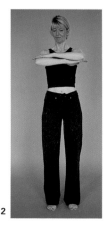

2

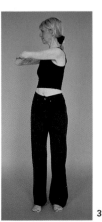

3

The body should stay centred, with the shoulders parallel to the floor

Keep your hips facing forward as you twist – the movement occurs in the upper body only

1. Stand with your legs hip-width apart, feet in parallel. Drop your shoulders and pull your shoulderblades down into your back. Lengthen up through the spine and back of the neck.

BENEFITS

- Stretches the waist and upper back
- Improves the posture
- Releases tension in the spine

2. Breathe in and bring your arms up to just below shoulder level, placing one forearm on top of the other, the fingers of one hand touching the elbow of the opposite arm, in a 'Cossack'-style pose. Do not hunch the shoulders as you bring the arms up.

3. Breathe out, lengthen up out of the waist and slowly twist round to the right with the upper body, making sure that the hips stay facing forwards. Keep the head in line with the shoulders – do not be tempted to take it any further round than the rest of the body. Twist as far as you can then breathe in and return to centre. Repeat for the other side. Repeat the sequence 5 to 10 times, trying to increase the twist each time.

CAUTION

- Do not twist round too far – twist from the waist, keeping the head in line with the body.
- If you suffer from a back problem, seek medical advice before attempting this exercise.

Chest Opener

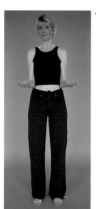

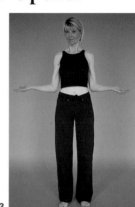

Make sure that you keep your shoulders down and your elbows tucked in to your waist throughout this exercise

BENEFITS

- Improves posture
- Works the upper arms and shoulders
- Releases tension at the base of the neck and across the tops of the shoulders
- Opens the chest

1. Stand with your back in neutral and your feet in parallel, hip-width apart, your spine and neck lengthened and your arms resting by your sides. Your legs should be straight with your knees soft. Tuck your elbows into your waist, and raise your hands up to waist level, palms facing upwards. Focus your eyes straight ahead in front of you.

2. Breathe out, contracting the abdominals, dropping the shoulders and drawing the shoulderblades down into your back.

3. Breathe in and take your hands slowly out to the sides and back as far as possible. Keep dropping your shoulders and drawing your shoulderblades down and back as you do this. Breathe out and slowly bring your hands back to centre. Repeat 5 to 10 times, moving the hands at an even pace, in time with the breath.

OPTION

This exercise can be done either sitting or standing. If you wish to sit, position yourself forward on the chair and place your feet hip-width apart on the floor in front of you. Make sure that your spine is in neutral with your spine and neck lengthened.

Push Up

3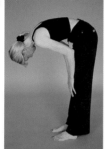

This is a flowing movement that should be done slowly and evenly, using a controlled movement

Keep your lower abdominals contracted to focus the strengthening effect of the move and provide support for your lower back

5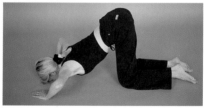

BENEFITS

- Strengthens the abdominals, the lower back, the upper body and the arms

1. Stand in neutral with feet hip-width apart and knees soft, your weight evenly distributed over both feet. Breathe in and contract your lower abdominals.

2. Breathe out, drop your head forward and start to roll down through the spine, vertebra by vertebra, using a slow, controlled movement.

3. Continue to roll down as you exhale, pausing to take an extra breath if you need to. As you roll, allow your hands to come to rest lightly on your knees.

4. When you have gone as far as you are comfortably able, bend your knees and place your hands onto the floor, fingertips first. Focus your eyes straight down at the floor and keep lengthening through the neck. Breathe in, then breathe out and walk your hands forward away from your body, gently dropping to your knees as you do so, until you are on all fours, with your knees directly below your hips and your hands directly below your shoulders.

5. Breathe in and, using a slow, even movement, breathe out and lower your upper body down the floor, sending your elbows out away from the body, and then push back up. Keep your abdominals contracted and your hips level. Repeat this push up 5 to 10 times, exhaling as you lower and inhale as you raise. To finish, breathe in, then breathe out as you walk your hands back, take your weight onto your feet and slowly roll back up to standing, bringing your head up last.

LYING-DOWN EXERCISES

Spine Curls

Keep the hips level, in line with the shoulders, and the knees stable throughout this exercise

Use a slow, controlled movement

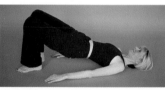

2

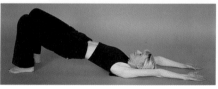

4

BENEFITS

- Increases flexibility in the spine
- Strengthens muscles in abdominal and pelvic areas
- Improves muscle control

1. Lie on your back with feet hip-width apart, knees bent, feet flat on the floor, heels as close to your body as possible, and arms resting by your sides. Lengthen through the spine and along the back of the neck.

2. Breathing out, contract the abdominals and tilt the pelvis up slightly, keeping the spine in contact with the floor. Breathe in and release, then breathe out, tilt the pelvis raising it slightly off the floor. Repeat, lifting the tailbone off the floor a little more each time, gradually peeling the spine away the floor, vertebra by vertebra. Breathe out as you lift and breathe in as you release the spine back down to the floor.

3. Breathe out, contract the abdominals and roll the tailbone up off the floor until you are resting on your shoulders, with the body in a diagonal slope, keeping the spine in neutral. Breathe in. Breathe out as you contract the abdominals and roll the spine slowly back down to the starting position. Repeat 3 to 5 times.

4. Repeat step 3, but now, once you reach the diagonal position, breathe in and slowly raise the arms up over the head and down to the floor, then breathe out as you bring them back to the starting position. Breathe in, then breathe out as you roll down through the spine onto the floor. For a slightly harder option, keep the arms in position over your head as you breathe out and roll back down through the spine, then breathe in as you bring the arms back. Repeat 5 to 10 times.

Arm Circles

*Maintain the spine in the neutral
position and the abdominals
contracted throughout this sequence*

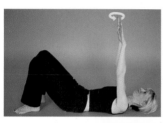

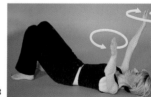

BENEFITS

- Strengthens the abdominal muscles
- Gently stretches and strengthens the arms
- Releases tension in the shoulders and chest

1. Lie on your back with your legs bent, ankles hip-width apart, feet flat on the floor. Place your arms by your sides. Drop the shoulders, drawing the shoulderblades down into your back. Check that the spine is in neutral. Breathe in, contracting the abdominals and bring the arms straight up to shoulder level, holding the hands shoulder-width apart, pointing straight up to the ceiling, palms facing away from you, towards your feet.

2. Breathe out, making small, slow circles with your arms, taking the arms up towards the head, around and out, then down and finally back up to the starting position. Breathe out as you take the arms up and away from the body, inhale as you bring them down and back in. Repeat 5 times using a smooth, even motion. Keep the arms and shoulders as relaxed as possible, elbows soft, with the shoulderblades drawn down into your back.

3. Repeat, changing the direction of the arm circles, exhaling as you take the hands down towards the body and out, then inhaling as you bring them up and round. Repeat 5 times. Change direction again and repeat the sequence one more time, making 5 circles in one direction and then 5 in the other. Once you are familiar with this exercise you can gradually make the circles bigger. If you have any tension in the shoulders, try sliding the arms along the floor as you bring the arms down and round.

Hip Rolls

As you rotate the hips in one direction and the head in the other, make sure you keep both shoulders in contact with the floor at all times

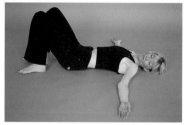

2

Use the abdominals to control the move as you roll: don't simply allow the weight of the legs to pull you over

CAUTION

Don't force this stretch – as you increase the rotation each time, only take it as far as is comfortable for you. As you develop flexibility in the spine and strength in the abdominal core you will automatically find you will gradually be able to take the stretch further.

1. Lie on your back in neutral, your legs bent, knees hip-width apart and pointing up to the ceiling, feet in parallel. Place your arms out to the sides with palms facing upwards. Breathe in and lengthen along the spine and back of the neck and relax the body, allowing the floor to support your weight.

BENEFITS

- Stretches the spine and waist muscles
- Relieves tightness and stiffness in the lower back
- Gently stretches the neck and releases tension

2. Breathe out, contract the abdominals and let your knees roll gently over to one side very slightly (the knees should move just a few inches to start with). At the same time rotate the head in the opposite direction.

3. Breathe in, contract the abdominals and breathe out as you bring the knees back to the starting position. Repeat on the other side.

4. Repeat the sequence a total of 5 to 10 times, taking the knees a little further over each time. As you start to rotate the hips further, allow the hip to lift up as you peel the lower back away from the floor vertebra by vertebra. As you bring the knees back to centre, let the spine roll slowly back down one vertebra at a time.

OPTION

Once you have developed strength and control in the abdominal core, you can try doing this exercise using the following position: float your legs up, one at a time, until they are at right-angles with the body (knees bent and shins parallel to the floor) and place a tennis ball or small cushion between your knees, to help stabilise the legs, then rotate the hips and the head as described above.

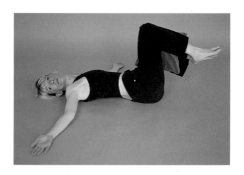

The Hundred

1. Lie on the floor with your legs bent, knees pointing up to the ceiling, feet parallel, and your arms by your sides with palms facing downwards.

2. Check that your spine is in neutral with your hips level and your eyes focussed up to the ceiling. Breathe in, then, as you breathe out, contract your abdominals and float your right leg up until the shin is parallel to the floor, with the knee at right angles. Holding the leg in this position and keeping the hips stable, drop the shoulders and lengthen the arms, lifting and lowering them in a fairly fast pumping action, 5 times for each in breath and 5 times for each out breath. Once you have reached 50 arm pumps, change legs and repeat for the other side.

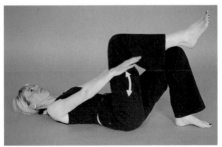

2

TIPS

There are several developments to this exercise, at various levels of difficulty. Choose an option that suits your current strength and ability. Remember, you will gain far more by working at a less demanding option while maintaining control and alignment, than by struggling with an exercise that is too difficult for you.

OPTION 1

If you already have good strength in your abdominal muscles, you can try this option. As you breathe out, extend the leg, lowering it slightly. Think of lengthening away from the hip, down the leg and out through the foot. Check that your spine is still in neutral with your abdominals contracted slightly. Holding this position, pump the arms as described above.

OPTION 2

This option increases the intensity of the exercise in the abdominal area. Breathe out and lower the extended leg a little closer to the floor. Holding this position, pump the arms as described above.

OPTION 3

Adopt the position described in step 1 above, then breathe in and release your lower back into the floor (this is sometimes referred to as 'imprinting'). Breathe out as you contract your lower abdominals floating

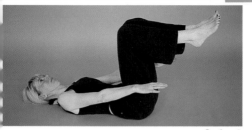

Option 3

your legs up, one after the other, until the
shins are parallel to the floor, with the knees at right
angles. Pump the arms as described above.

OPTION 4

Once you have improved your strength and stability
you are ready for this difficult option (shown below).
Follow the instructions for option 3 then, once you
have raised both legs to the right-angle position,
breathe in and then breathe out, squeeze the inner
thighs together, and extend both legs out and lower
them down towards the floor. At the same time drop
your chin to your chest
and raise your head off the
ground. Pump the arms as
described above, then
breathe in as you return
the legs to the right-angle
position then lower them
to the floor, one at a time.

BENEFITS

• Strengthens the
  abdominal core
• Muscle control
• Builds stamina

Neck Pull

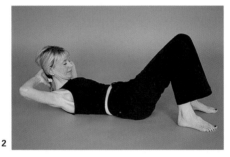

2

Keep the abdominals contracted and the pelvis tucked under to avoid any pressure or strain on the lower back.

BENEFITS

- Strengthens the abdominal muscles
- Stretches the neck, shoulders and upper back
- Increases the flexibility of the spine

1. Lie on your back with your spine in neutral and your legs slightly apart, knees bent. Place your hands behind your head, point your elbows out away from the body. Drop your shoulders and draw your shoulderblades down into your back.

2. Breathe in, lengthen your neck and drop your chin onto your chest very slightly. Breathe out as you contract the abdominals, then slowly raise your head and begin rolling up through the spine. Curl your shoulders away from the floor, vertebra by vertebra, keeping your shoulders down. When you begin to feel resistance in the abdominals, pause, breathe in, then breathe out, increasing the contraction in the abdominals, tilt the pelvis forward, and slowly roll back down to the starting position. Repeat 5 to 10 times.

OPTION

When you have developed sufficient strength in the abdominals and flexibility in the spine, try repeating the move with your legs extended, knees and ankles together. Roll up to through the spine until you reach a sitting position. Continue the movement, breathing in, contracting the abdominals, then breathing out, and curling forward as far as you can. As you stretch forward, imagine rounding your upper body up and over a large beach ball. Inhale and roll back down to the floor. Repeat 5 to 10 times.

Neck Stretch

This should be a smooth, slow, gentle stretch of the neck muscles – avoid making any jerky movements or forcing the stretch too far

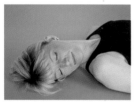

Keep the head on the floor as you move

2

Keep the jaw relaxed – make sure you are not clenching your teeth

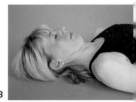

3

If you are uncomfortable lying on the floor, place a small cushion under your head

1. Lie on the floor with your back in neutral, your legs bent, knees hip-width apart and pointing up to the ceiling, feet in parallel. Place your arms by your sides with palms down. Breathe in, soften through the chest area, lengthen along the spine and back of the neck and let the weight of your body sink into the floor.

BENEFITS

- Releases tension and stiffness in the neck
- Stretches neck muscles
- Improves posture
- Eases neck and upper-shoulder pain

2. Breathe out and contract the abdominal muscles very slightly then allow your head to roll slowly over to one side, keeping the neck lengthened and the head in contact with the floor. Think of rotating the head and taking the ear towards the floor. Breathe in and bring the head slowly back to centre, then exhale as you roll the head to the other side. Repeat the sequence 5 to 10 times.

3. Starting from the centre position, breathe out and slowly tuck the chin towards the chest, lengthening and stretching the neck. Breathe in as you gently release the chin back up to centre. Repeat 5 to 10 times.

CAUTION

If you experience any pain, stop immediately and seek medical advice.

Single Leg Stretch

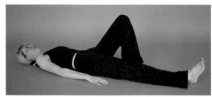

2

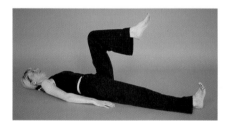

Option 1

BENEFITS

- Strengthens the abdominal core
- Works the hip flexors, strengthening and improving flexibility

1. Lie on your back with your legs bent, knees pointing up to the ceiling, feet in parallel. Place your arms by your sides with palms down.

2. Keeping your spine in neutral and your hips stable, in line with your shoulders, breathe in, contract the abdominals, then exhale and extend the right leg, sliding your heel along the ground. Inhale as you slide your leg back to the starting position. Repeat for the left leg. Repeat, alternating the legs, for a total of 10 to 20 repetitions.

OPTION 1

1. Once you can confidently extend the legs while keeping the abdominals contracted, the spine in neutral and the hips level, you are ready to try floating the left leg up until the shin is parallel to the floor, knee at right angles. Hold the leg in this position and extend the right leg out, as described in step 1.

2. Breathe in and draw the extended leg back to the starting position, then exhale as you float the raised leg back down to the ground. Repeat for the other side. Repeat 5 to 10 times on each side, making sure the raised leg is kept at right angles and the hips stable.

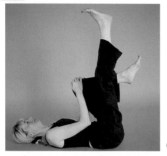

Option 2

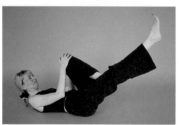

Option 3

OPTION 2

1. In this version, float both legs up to towards your chest, one at a time, knees bent. Rest your hands on the outside of your knees, elbows pointing out.

2. Breathe in and contract the abdominals, then breathe out and extend the right leg up to the

ceiling, placing both hands either side of your left
knee as you do so. Breathe in as you bring your
right leg back in to your chest. Repeat 5 to 10 times,
using alternating legs.

OPTION 3

1. As the strength and control in your abdominal
   muscles gradually increases, you can try bringing the
   extended leg closer to the floor. This will intensify
   the effect of the exercise on the abdominal core.
   Float both legs up to towards your chest, one at a
   time, knees bent. Rest your hands on the outside of
   your knees, elbows pointing outwards. At the same
   time, drop your chin to your chest slightly, and raise
   your head up away from the floor, lengthening
   through the neck as you do so. Keep your shoulders
   down and away from your ears, and your
   shoulderblades pulled down into your back

2. Breathe in and contract the abdominals, then
   breathe out and extend the right leg out, placing
   both hands either side of your left knee as you do
   so. Breathe in as you bring your right leg back in to
   your chest. Breathe out as you extend the left leg,
   placing your hands on your right knee. Repeat the
   sequence 5 to 10 times, keeping the head up
   throughout.

Double Leg Stretch

*Maintain the spine in the neutral position
and the abdominals contracted throughout
this sequence*

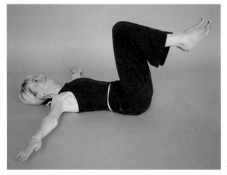

2

BENEFITS

- Strengthens the abdominal muscles
- Gently stretches and strengthens the arms
- Releases tension in the shoulders and chest

1. Lie on your back with legs bent, ankles hip-width apart and feet flat on the floor. Place your arms by your sides. Drop the shoulders, drawing the shoulder-blades down into your back. Check that the spine is in neutral. Breathe in and contract the abdominals. Keeping the spine in neutral, bring the arms straight up to shoulder level, holding the hands shoulder-width apart, fingers pointing straight to the ceiling, palms facing away from you towards your feet.

2. Breathe out and float the legs up, one at a time, until the shins are parallel to the floor, with the knees at right angles. Holding the legs in this position, breathe in, then breathe out and start circling the arms, taking them up towards the head, around and out, then down and finally back up to the starting position. Breathe out as you take the arms up and away from the body, inhale as you bring them down and back in. Repeat 5 times using a smooth, even motion. Keep the arms and shoulders as relaxed as possible, elbows soft, with the shoulderblades drawn down into your back.

3. Breathe in, then breathe out and switch the direction of the arm circles, exhaling as you take the hands down towards the body and out, then inhaling as you bring them up and round. Repeat 5 times. Change direction again; repeat the sequence one more time, circling 5 times in one direction and then 5 in the other. To finish, inhale and lower the arms first, then float the legs back down to the floor, one at a time.

OPTION

When you are familiar with the above sequence and have developed sufficient strength in the abdominal core, try extending the legs out at a 45-degree angle to the floor as you circle the arms. Lower the legs towards the floor if you want to work the abdominals harder, but make sure that you are able to keep the spine in neutral and the hips stable as you do so. Raise the legs up towards the ceiling for a slightly easier option.

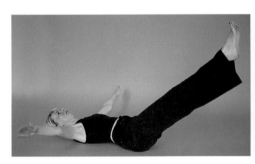

Hamstring Stretch

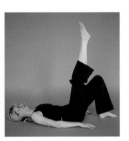

This stretch can be done with your hands grasping the thigh of the extended leg or, for more intensity, with a stretchy exercise band (or small towel) held over the foot

1

Make sure your hips stay level and in contact with the floor as you stretch

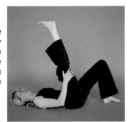

2

CAUTION

Do not arch the back as you stretch – keep it in neutral and contract the abdominals to support your lower back.

BENEFITS

- Stretches and strengthens the hamstrings
- Gently stretches the gluteals and the lower back
- Releases tension in the legs and lower back

1. Lie on your back with your spine in neutral, legs bent, knees hip-width apart and your feet parallel. Breathe in and lengthen along the back and neck. Breathe out as you contract the abdominals and lift the right leg to a 90-degree angle, with toes pointed.

2. Breathe in; place your hands around the right thigh. Breathe out and slowly pull the extended leg in towards you. Breathe in and release. Repeat 5 to 10 times, breathing out as you draw the leg in, breathing in as you release. Repeat for the other leg.

OPTION

Follow steps 1 and 2 above, first bringing the knee into the chest to place the exercise band over the foot and then extending the leg out, flexing the foot. Hold one end of the band in each hand, resting your upper arms and elbows on the floor. Breathe out, contract the abdominals and pull down on the band to increase the hamstring stretch. Breathe in and release. Keep the shoulders down and the shoulderblades drawn down into your back. Repeat the stretch 5 to 10 times, breathing out as you stretch, breathing in as you release. Repeat for the other leg.

One Leg Circles

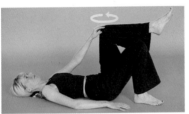

2

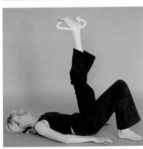

Option

Imagine the circles as coming from the hip joint, rather than the knees, encouraging the hip joint to release as you keep circling

BENEFITS

- Strengthens the pelvic and abdominal muscles
- Stretches and strengthens the legs
- Improves flexibility in the legs and hip

1. Lie on your back, with your spine in the neutral position, your knees bent and your feet flat on the floor in front of you, approximately hip-width apart.

2. Breathe in, contract your abdominals and breathe out as you lift your left leg in to your chest, until the shin is parallel to the floor, with the knee at a right angle. Place the fingertips of your left hand on your raised knee. Breathe in.

3. Breathe out and, using your fingertips to guide you, circle your knee 5 to 10 times in one direction, and then 5 to 10 times in the other, pausing for a breath, and then breathing out again as you change direction. Make sure you keep the opposite leg still, with the knee pointing straight up towards the ceiling. Breathe in, then breathe out as you release the right leg back down to the floor. Repeat for the right leg.

OPTIONS

1. Once you can make controlled, smooth circles with your knee, you no longer need your hand to guide you – let it rest at your side. Gradually increase the size of the circles, maintaining a slow, even movement in time with the breathing.

2. To increase the difficulty, straighten the raised leg up towards the ceiling and draw the circles with your feet. Keep lengthening the leg out of the hip, away from the body. Keep the knee soft. Circle the leg 10 times in one direction, then in the other.

Shoulder Lifts

Relax your face and avoid tightening your jaw or clenching the teeth

Keep the shoulders dropped throughout and the neck and shoulders relaxed

3

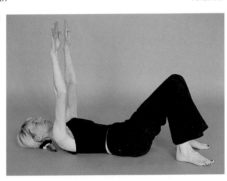

Continue to pull the shoulderblades down into the back, even as you lift the shoulder up away from the floor

---

BENEFITS

- Releases tension in neck, shoulders and upper back
- Gently mobilises the shoulder joints and stretches the arms
- Improves posture and reduces stress

CAUTION

Take care that you don't tense your neck as you reach upwards with the arms.

1. Lie on the floor with your back in the neutral position, your legs bent, knees hip-width apart and pointing up to the ceiling, feet in parallel. Rest your arms down by your sides with palms facing downwards. Breathe in as you relax and let the weight of your body sink into the floor as you lengthen along the spine and back of the neck.

2. Breathe out, contract the abdominals a little, keeping the back in neutral, and allow your arms to float up to the ceiling, in line with the shoulders. Keep the arms straight, the elbows soft and the fingers extended.

3. Breathe in and stretch one hand up towards the ceiling, allowing the shoulderblade to lift up away from the floor very slightly. Breathe out as you drop the shoulderblade back down to the floor, keeping the movement slow and controlled. Repeat, this time stretching the other hand up towards the ceiling.

4. Repeat the stretch 10 times (5 times on each side), using alternate arms.

5. Breath in as you lower the arms back down to your sides, keeping the shoulderblades pulled down into the back and the shoulders dropped.

Arm Openings

Keep the head in contact with the floor as you move

You may place a small cushion between your knees, to help you keep your pelvis stable and your knees in alignment

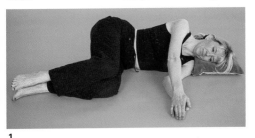

1

Move the upper body while keeping the lower body still. Only take the arm back as far as you can while maintaining the stability of the hips and legs

BENEFITS

- Mobilises and stretches the spine
- Reduces stiffness and tightness in the back
- Opens the chest area, gently stretching arms and neck and relieving tension

1. Lie on your left side with your knees bent up at right angles to your body, knees and ankles together. Your back should be in neutral, with the spine parallel to the floor – make sure that your waist is lifted slightly, and not dropped to the floor. Place a small cushion under your head to keep your neck in alignment. Position the arms straight out to the side, at just below shoulder level, one hand on top of the other.

2. Breathe in and lengthen the spine and neck, allowing your weight to sink into the floor, but keeping the back in the neutral position.

3. Breathe out, contract the abdominals and slowly raise the right hand up towards the ceiling then back behind you as far as possible, in a semicircular arc. Keep the arm straight and the elbow soft as you move. Follow the movement of the hand with the eyes, rotating the head and gently stretching the muscles of the neck.

4. Breathe in as you slowly bring the arm back to the starting position, making sure you keep the abdominals contracted and again following the movement of the hand with the eyes. Keep lengthening through the neck as you move.

5. Repeat 5 times on this side, then switch positions and repeat the sequence 5 times lying on the right side.

Make sure both shoulders remain in contact with the floor as you slowly stretch the arm

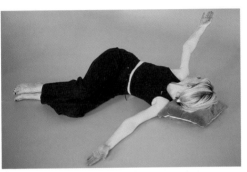

3

CAUTION

Do not attempt this exercise if you suffer from any back or neck problems or have sustained an injury to the back or neck. If in doubt, consult a doctor.

Windmill

Keep the eyes focussed up to the ceiling

Maintain the spine in the neutral position and the abdominals contracted throughout this sequence

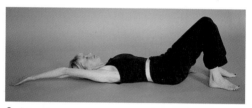

2

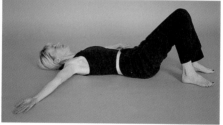

3

Once you have mastered this exercise, practise changing direction with each rotation

BENEFITS

- Mobilises the muscles of the shoulder area
- Gently stretches and strengthens the arms
- Improves co-ordination

1. Lie on your back with your legs bent, ankles hip-width apart, feet flat on the floor. Place your arms by your sides. Drop the shoulders, drawing the shoulderblades down into your back. Check that the spine is in neutral. Breathe in, contracting the abdominals, and float the arms up to shoulder level, with the hands shoulder-width apart, pointing straight up to the ceiling, palms facing away from you, fingers extended.

2. Breathe out, taking the right arm up behind your head, palm up, and the left arm down to your side, palm down.

3. In a continuous, even movement, circle the right arm out to the side, down towards your feet and then back up to the starting position at the same time as you circle the left arm out to the side and round towards your head, then up towards the ceiling, back to the starting position. Keep circling the arms for 5 to 10 rotations, breathing out as you take the arms down towards the floor and out to the sides, then breathing in as you bring the arms back to centre.

4. Change the direction of the arms and repeat the sequence.

The Corkscrew

CAUTION

This requires a strong abdominal core and good muscle control, and should only be attempted once you have developed sufficient strength to keep control even when the move requires you to twist off-centre.

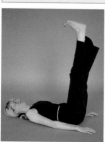

4

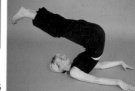

5

BENEFITS

- Improves balance
- Builds strength
- Develops muscle control

1. Lie on your back with your legs stretched straight out in front of you, toes pointing away, knees and ankles together. Rest your arms by your sides, palms to the floor. Check that your spine is in neutral and breathe in.

2. Breathe out as you contract the abdominals and tilt the pelvis forward slightly, tucking the tailbone in. Continue to breathe as you raise your legs up towards the ceiling, keeping the spine in neutral.

3. Using the abdominal contraction to control the lift, squeeze the inner thighs together as you raise your legs, bringing them up and over your head, and slowly peeling the spine away from the floor, one vertebra at a time.

4. Take your legs over behind your head, as far down to the floor as you can, and continue curling up the spine until your weight is resting your shoulders. Press down with your hands to stabilise yourself, if necessary. Keep the legs straight and the knees soft.

5. Keeping legs and hips in parallel, breathe in, then breathe out, increase the contraction in the abdominals and slowly draw a circle in the air with the feet, moving them around to the right, then around and down, across, and around and up to the left. Breathe in then breathe out and draw a circle in the opposite direction. Repeat this 'corkscrew' movement 5 to 10 times. To finish, breathe in as you bring the legs back to centre; breathe out as you lower them to the floor.

Jack Knife

To maximise the strength-building effect of this exercise, roll down through the spine as slowly as possible, controlling the movement throughout using the abdominal muscles

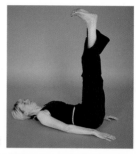

2

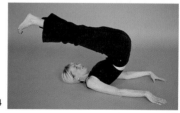

4

BENEFITS

- Builds strength
- Improves muscle control
- Stretches the back, shoulder and arm muscles

CAUTION

- Before you attempt this exercise make sure you have developed sufficient strength in the abdominals and flexibility in the spine. To strengthen your abdominals and muscle control, practise the Rolling Up exercise described on pages 98–9.

- Do not attempt this exercise if you have any history of neck or back problems. If you are in any doubt, seek medical advice.

- As you roll up, keep the weight of the body on the shoulders and avoid rolling onto the neck.

1. Lie on your back with your legs extended, feet pointed, knees and ankles together. Let your arms rest by your sides, palms facing downwards. Pull the shoulderblades down and back, making sure the spine is in neutral with the back of the neck lengthened. Focus the eyes straight up at the ceiling.

2. Breathe in, then breathe out as you contract the abdominals and tilt the pelvis forwards. Continuing to breathe out, squeeze the buttocks, squeeze the inner thighs together and lift your feet up towards the ceiling, keeping your legs straight, knees soft and toes pointed.

3. Still using the outbreath, continue the movement lowering your feet a few inches behind your head, taking them straight down towards the floor, and

allow your tailbone and lower spine to peel away from the floor, vertebra by vertebra. If necessary, press down with your hands and use your arms to help you balance.

4. When you have gone as far as you can while controlling the move with the abdominal core, breathe in and slowly roll back down through the spine and then lower the legs. Make sure you maintain the abdominal contraction as you roll back down, working against gravity and keeping the movement as slow and controlled as possible. Repeat 5 to 10 times.

OPTION

Once you have completely mastered the above move, you are ready to challenge yourself a little further. Follow the above instructions, this time continuing to peel the spine up away from the floor on the outbreath, until your body and legs are in a line pointing straight up towards the ceiling with your weight resting on your shoulders, neck and arms. The aim here is to control the entire movement with the abdominal core, but, if you need to, use your arms to stabilise yourself. Breathe in and roll back down through the spine to the starting position, keeping the movement slow and controlled. To guide you, try to keep your feet positioned directly above your face for as long as possible as you roll down through the spine. Repeat 5 to 10 times.

Teaser

BENEFITS

- Builds strength in the abdominal core
- Improves muscle control and stability
- Increases strength and flexibility in the spine

The aim here is to work the upper body without using the legs and arms to help you

Keep the movement smooth and controlled as you slowly raise and lower the body

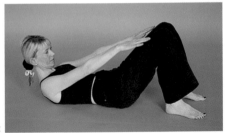

2

Keep dropping the shoulders and drawing the shoulderblades down into your back throughout the entire sequence

Make sure the legs remain still and in position as you roll up and down through the spine

CAUTION

If you feel any pain or discomfort in your lower back, stop immediately and seek medical advice.

1. Lie on your back with your legs bent, knees hip-width apart and pointing up to the ceiling, feet in parallel. Place your arms by your sides with palms down. Lengthen along the spine and back of the neck.

2. Breathe out, contract the abdominals, and float the hands up towards the ceiling until the arms are parallel to the thighs. At the same time, drop the chin slightly towards the chest and start to roll slowly up through the spine, one vertebra at a time, as far as you can, controlling the move with the abdominals. Keep the shoulders relaxed and the shoulderblades pulled down into your back.

3. Breathe in, contract the abdominals and roll slowly back down through the spine to the floor. Repeat 5 to 10 times.

OPTION 1

Once you are comfortable with the movement, try the sequence keeping one foot on the ground, knee bent, as above, and extending the other leg upwards, squeezing the inner thighs together as you roll up through the spine. Repeat 5 to 10 times, alternating the legs.

OPTION 2

Repeat the sequence given above, but this time, extend both legs. Keep squeezing the inner thighs together and lengthening the legs away from you as you roll through the spine. If you start to feel your back arching, then raise the legs up towards the ceiling a little, until you feel comfortable once more.

OPTION 3

Once you have mastered the above technique, try beginning the exercise from a sitting position, extending both legs then lightly grasping the backs of the knees as you slowly roll down through the spine, vertebra by vertebra, as far as you can, keeping the alignment and using the abdominal muscles to control the movement. Breathe in as you roll back up to sitting. Repeat 5 to 10 times, keeping legs raised throughout.

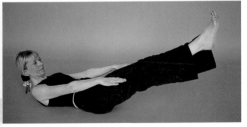

Option 2

Scissors

BENEFITS

- Builds strength in the abdominal core, back and legs
- Improves concentration and breath control
- Increases flexibility

Keep the shoulders down and the shoulderblades pulled down into your back throughout this move

3

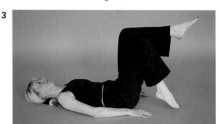

Focus on contracting the abdominal muscles, keeping the spine in neutral and the hips level as you 'scissor'

As you move the legs, think of lengthening them away from you, out of the hip joint

CAUTION

If you feel any pain or discomfort in your lower back or neck, stop immediately and seek medical advice.

1. Lie on the floor with knees bent, hip-width apart, feet parallel, and arms by your sides. Breathe in, checking that your spine is in neutral and your neck and shoulders relaxed.

2. Breathe out, contract the abdominals and float your legs up, one at a time, knees bent, until the thighs are at right angles to the body and shins parallel to the floor.

3. Breathe in, keeping your legs in this position, then breathe out and, still keeping the knees bent, 'dip' the toes of one foot down towards the floor, as if into a pool of water, breathe in as you bring the leg back to centre. Repeat 5 to 10 times using alternate legs. You do not need to take the foot all the way to the floor at first – just take it as far as you can while keeping your spine in neutral, your hips level and your abdominals contracted. As you progress you will gradually be able to take the movement further.

OPTION

As your abdominal strength and muscle control develop, gradually extend the legs, increasing the angle of the knee bend little by little, until you are able to do the exercise with completely straight legs, taking one down towards the floor as the other one lifts up. At the same time, tuck your chin in to your chest slightly and lengthen along the back of the neck, bringing your head and shoulders up away from the floor. Raise and lower the legs at a controlled, even pace in time with the breathing, changing the breath as you change the direction of the legs. Repeat 5 to 10 times on each leg.

Rolling Up

BENEFITS

- Strengthens the abdominals
- Mobilises and strengthens the back
- Improves muscle control

Concentrate on keeping the movement slow, flowing and even

Use the abdominal contraction to control the move

Keep your knees bent and feet on the floor

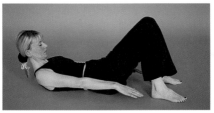

2

Don't worry if you can't roll up very far to start with, the important element is for you to work the abdominals keeping the body in the correct alignment. Over time, as you develop and strengthen, your range of movement will automatically increase

CAUTION

Avoid this exercise if you suffer from neck problems.

1. Lie on your back with knees bent, feet flat on the floor hip-width apart. Put your arms by your sides. Drop the shoulders, drawing the shoulderblades down into your back. Check that your spine is in neutral.

2. Breathe in, contract the abdominals, tuck the chin into the chest slightly, lengthen along the back of the neck and allow the head to curl up from the floor. Raise your arms an inch off the floor, lengthening them away from you, fingers extended, as you begin to roll up. Keep the shoulders dropped and the shoulderblades pulled down into your back as you roll up through the spine, vertebra by vertebra.

3. When you start to feel resistance in the abdominals and can roll up no further, pause, breathe in, contract the abdominals, then breathe out as you slowly roll back down to the floor, controlling the movement with the abdominals. Repeat 5 to 10 times.

OPTION

As an alternative, begin from the sitting position, with your knees bent and your feet flat on the floor in a parallel position. Grasp your thighs with your hands, arms relaxed. Breathe in, contract the abdominals, tilt your pelvis forward slightly and slowly curl back, rolling down through the spine. When you feel the point of resistance in the abdominals, breathe in and return to an upright position. Repeat 5 to 10 times, keeping your eyes focussed straight in front of you as you curl.

Leg Lifts

BENEFITS

- Strengthens and lengthens the leg muscles
- Tones and strengthens the buttocks, hips and thighs
- Mobilises the hip joint
- Develops the abdominal core
- Improves muscle control

TIPS

- As your legs grow stronger, you may add light leg weights to increase the intensity of the stretches.
- Keep your back aligned and your spine parallel to the floor – do not allow the waist to drop to the floor as you work the legs.
- Relax the head and neck, allowing the arm (and cushion) to support it.
- Lengthen the lower arm away from you as you work.

CAUTION

- Do not arch your back as you work – concentrate on keeping the spine in neutral and the back long.
- Keep contracting the abdominals to support your lower back.

These exercises can be performed as a sequence: complete the lifts, circles and pulses for one leg before changing position and repeating on the other side.

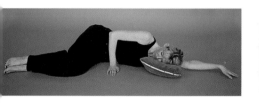

Single Leg Lifts

1. Lie on your left side with your left arm extended away from you and your head resting on your arm. Place a small cushion or folded towel under your head to keep your neck in line with your spine. Bend your knees up to form a right-angle with your body and place your right hand, palm down, on the floor in front of your chest to help you balance. Focus your eyes straight out in front of you. Breathe in.

2. Breathe out, contract the abdominals and extend the right leg, lengthening it away from you, out of the hip joint. Keep the foot flexed as you lengthen down the back of the leg and out through the heel. Allow the leg to lift from the floor as you lengthen, but keep the extended leg low – aim to raise it just

an inch or so away from the ground. Do not arch your back or let your waist drop to the floor.

3. Breathe in and lower the leg, keeping it straight and in line with the body.

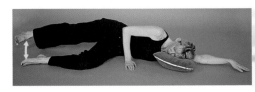

4. Breathe out and extend the leg once more. Repeat 5 to 10 times. To finish, breathe in, then breathe out, contract the abdominals and lower the right leg, bending it back up to rest on top of the left leg.

5. Change your position and repeat the sequence for the left leg.

Leg Circles

1. Follow the instructions for step 1 above.

2. Breathe out, contract the abdominals and extend the right leg away from you, so that it is in line with your hips, parallel to the floor.

3. Holding this position and keeping your breathing slow and even, make small, controlled circles

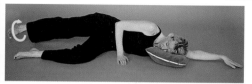

(approximately the size of a coconut) with your leg. Circle 5 to 10 times in one direction and then 5 to 10 times in the other, lengthening the leg away from you, out of the hip joint, as you circle. Again, flex the foot as you lengthen down the back of the leg and out through the heel.

4. Breathe in, then breathe out and lower the right leg, bending the knee and bringing it back to rest on the left leg.

5. Change your position and repeat for the left leg.

Leg Pulses

1. Follow the instructions as steps 1 and 2 of the Leg Circles exercise above.

2. Breathe out and 'pulse' the extended leg down an inch or two and then back up again – do not raise it higher than the level of your hips.

3. Pulse the leg 10 to 20 times in total, changing the breathing every 5 counts.

4. Breathe in, then breathe out as you lower the leg back to the starting position.

5. Change your position and repeat for the left leg.

OPTION – LOWER LEG PULSES

1. Still lying on your left side with your left arm extended away from you, your head resting on your left arm and your right hand on the floor in front of you to help you balance and your knees bent up at right angles, place a cushion under your right knee to raise it slightly off the ground and prevent you from tilting your hip forwards.

2. Extend your left leg out along the ground at an angle of 45° to the body. Focus your eyes straight out in front of you. Breathe in.

3. Breathe out, contract your abdominals and pulse the left leg up away from the ground a total of 10 to 20 times, changing the breath every 5 counts as before.

4. Breathe in and bend your left leg back to join your right leg.

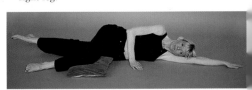

5. Change your position and repeat for the right leg.

OPTION – ARM POSITION

Once you have developed sufficient stability, muscle control and strength in the abdominal core, try resting your uppermost arm along the side of the body as you perform these leg exercises: if you start to wobble, or lose your balance, place your hand back down on the floor in front of you – you are not yet ready for this variation.

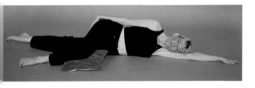

OPTION – LEG POSITION

When you have mastered the above leg-lift sequence, keeping the bottom leg bent up at a right-angle, try making this sequence of exercises a little more challenging by extending the bottom leg along the floor, in line with the body. You will need to work harder to keep control and stability in this position. If you find you are struggling and unable to maintain the correct alignment, return to the previous version.

Double Leg Lifts (Side)

BENEFITS

- Works the abdominals, the hips, the buttocks and the leg muscles
- Increases strength
- Improves muscle control

Avoid tilting the shoulder or hip forward as you extend and raise the legs

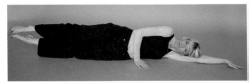

3

Concentrate on keeping your back in the neutral position as you raise the legs away from the floor

1. Lie on your left side with your body in a straight line, knees and ankles together. Rest your left arm along the floor, to support the head. (Place a small cushion under your head to support it, if you prefer.) Position the right arm along the side of your body, or, if you need, place your right hand on the floor in front of you to help you balance.

2. Check that your spine is in neutral with your shoulders and hips aligned. Lift your waist up away from the floor to keep the spine in its correct alignment. Breathe in.

3. Breathe out, contract the abdominals and, keeping your knees and ankles together, squeeze the inner thighs together and slowly extend both legs, allowing them to raise up away from the floor. Make sure that your legs remain in line with the body. The toes should be softly pointed.

4. Breathe in and lower the legs, but do not bring them all the way back down to the floor. Repeat 5 to 10 times. Change position and repeat for the other side.

OPTION

To increase the intensity of the movement, breathe out as you raise the legs, then hold this position and breathe in, then breathe out as you lower the legs.

Inner Thigh Stretch

Stay centred and avoid rolling to one side or the other as you stretch

Keep the tailbone in contact with the floor and allow the weight of the legs to create the initial stretch, releasing through the hips

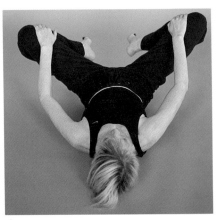

2

BENEFITS

- Stretches the inner thigh muscles
- Releases tension in the lower back, hips and pelvic area
- Rebalances the pelvis

1. Lie on your back with your knees bent. Inhale and lengthen through the spine and neck. Float your legs up, one at a time, keeping your knees bent. Rest your hands on your knees and let the knees drop out to the sides. Inhale and lengthen along the spine and neck, dropping your shoulders away from your ears and drawing the shoulderblades down and back behind you.

2. Breathe out, contract the abdominals and gently pull the knees apart, increasing the stretch to the inner thighs. Inhale and release. Repeat this stretch 5 to 10 times, increasing the stretch little by little each time. Breathe out as you stretch the legs apart and breathe in as you release.

CAUTION

Do not pull the knees too far out to the sides – let gravity do most of the work for you.

Rolling Over

BENEFITS

- Improves the flexibility of the spine
- Strengthening the abdominals
- Increases muscle control
- Stretches the hamstring, shoulder and neck areas

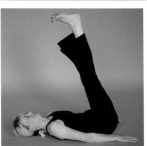

Avoid this exercise if you suffer from any neck or lower-back problems

3

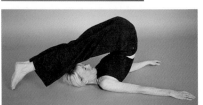

5

1. Lie on your back with your knees bent, feet flat on the floor, hip-width apart, and your spine in neutral. Rest your arms by your sides, palms facing down.

2. Breathe in, then breathe out, contract the abdominals and float the legs up, one at a time, keeping the knees at right-angles to the body, shins parallel to the floor. Breathe in.

3. Breathe out and slowly lower your feet straight down towards your face as far as possible, keeping your spine on the floor.

4. Continue the movement as you exhale, taking your feet over behind your head, allowing the spine to peel away from the floor, one vertebra at a time. If necessary, press down into the floor with your arms to stabilise yourself. Don't worry if you are unable to take your feet all the way to the floor at this stage, just take them as far as you can, trying to increase the stretch a little more each time. When you have reached as far as you can, breathe in.

5. Breathe out, contract the abdominals and start to roll slowly back down through the spine, vertebra by vertebra. Use the abdominal muscles to control the move as you work against gravity and roll back down. Bend the knees a little if you find it too hard to keep your legs straight for this section of the movement.

6. Once your tailbone is in contact with the floor, bring the legs back so that the feet are pointing straight up to the ceiling. Repeat the sequence 5 to 10 times.

Ankle Circles

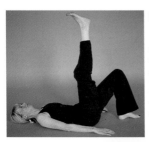

2

These exercises can be performed lying down or in a sitting position

Keep your breathing slow and even as you carry out this exercise

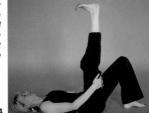

4

BENEFITS

- Strengthens and stretches the ankles
- Relieves tired feet and legs
- Improves circulation in the legs

1. Lie on your back with your legs bent, knees pointing up to the ceiling, feet in parallel.

2. Keeping your spine in neutral and your hips level and in line with your shoulders, breathe in, contract the abdominals, then exhale and float the right leg upwards, bending your knee in towards your chest and extending the right foot up towards the ceiling. Check that your ankle is in line with your hip and that you have not taken the leg out too far or in towards the centre.

3. Grasp your right thigh with both hands, to make sure that the leg remains still as you flex and rotate the feet. Bend your arms and point your elbows out to the sides.

4. Slowly flex your right foot in towards your face then release it back, making the entire movement as smooth as possible. Repeat 5 to 10 times.

5. Now, maintaining this position, circle the foot 5 to 10 times in one direction, then 5 to 10 times in the opposite direction.

6. Breathe out, contract your abdominals and lower your right foot back down to the floor.

7. Repeat the sequence for the left leg.

Squeezing The Pillow

This is an excellent exercise to use at the end of your routine

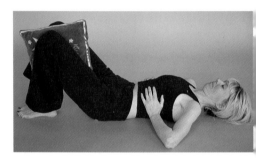

BENEFITS

- Strengthens the inner thighs
- Improves pelvic alignment
- Releases tension in the lower back and buttocks

TIPS

- Maintain the back in neutral as you squeeze, keeping the tailbone in contact with the floor.
- Keep the ribs down as you squeeze – placing your hands on your ribs will allow you to check that you are not lifting them.
- Make sure that your neck and shoulders are relaxed and that you are not clenching your jaw.
- Focus on squeezing the knees together – do not tighten the buttocks or the hip area.
- Once you are confident that you can squeeze without lifting the ribs, then position the arms at your sides, palms down.

1. Lie on your back with your knees bent, feet flat on the floor, knees and ankles together. Place a cushion or pillow between your knees. Rest your hands on your ribs with your elbows pointing out to the side. Breathe in.

2. Breathe out, contract the abdominals and squeeze the cushion with your knees. Hold for a count of ten, continuing to breathe out as you squeeze. Breathe in and release. Repeat 5 times.

EXERCISES LYING ON FRONT

Horizontal Star

Keep the neck lengthened throughout the entire sequence

4

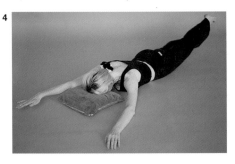

Do not raise the legs or arms too high off the ground – think of lengthening them out of the hip and shoulder joints, rather than lifting them

Make sure you keep both hips on the floor and the pelvis stable as you extend the legs

CAUTION

Keep the abdominals contracted as you stretch, to protect your lower back.

1. Lie face down on the floor, with a small cushion under your forehead for support, if you prefer. Your legs and arms should be slightly wider than hip- or shoulder-width apart so that you are lying on the floor in a 'star' position.

2. Drop your shoulders down away from your ears and pull your shoulderblades down into your back.

3. Breathe in and lengthen along the spine and neck.

4. Breathe out, contract the abdominals and lengthen the right arm and the left leg, raising them off the ground very slightly and keeping the elbows soft as you stretch.

5. Breathe in and release back down, then repeat for the other arm and leg.

6. Repeat the sequence 5 to 10 times, using opposite arms and legs each time and alternating with each repetition.

Shoulder Press

*This exercise works the upper back and shoulders
without involving the muscles of the lower body –
allow the legs and buttocks to stay relaxed and soft as
you raise and lower the upper body*

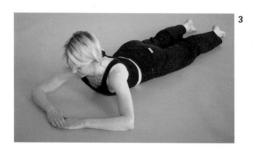

3

*Work both sides of
the body evenly,
keeping shoulders
and hips parallel
to each other as
you raise and
lower the upper
body evenly*

*If you regularly spend
time at a computer,
behind a desk or behind
the wheel of a vehicle,
take a few minutes a
day to carry out this
exercise – you will feel
the benefits almost
immediately*

BENEFITS

- Strengthens the upper back
- Releases tension in the neck and shoulders
- Improves posture and alignment
- Increases muscle control

1. Lie on your front with your legs straight, knees and ankles slightly apart, forehead resting on the floor, your hands placed, one on top of each other, slightly above your head, elbows pointing out to the sides. Lengthen along the spine and the back of the neck. Breathe in.

2. Breathe out, contract the abdominals, drop the shoulders and pull the shoulderblades down into your back as you raise the upper body away from the floor, using the muscles of the upper back. Keep your hands in position on the floor, but do not push down on them as you raise up or use them to support you – you should be able to lift them off the floor without changing the position of your body.

3. Keeping your abdominals contracted, your shoulders dropped and your shoulderblades pulled down, breathe in and relax back down, resting your forehead back on the floor. Keep your spine and neck lengthened and the abdominals contracted. Repeat 5 times.

Dart

Work both sides of the body evenly, keeping your shoulders and hips parallel as you lift – avoid leaning to one side as you raise up

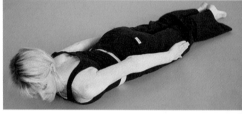

3

If necessary, place a small cushion on the floor, under your forehead, to keep the neck in line with the spine

BENEFITS

- Strengthens the upper back
- Releases tension in the neck and shoulders
- Improves posture and alignment
- Increases muscle control

1. Lie on your front with your legs straight, big toes together, heels dropped out to the sides. Rest your head on the floor, facing to one side. Place your arms by your sides, fingers extended downwards. Breathe in and lengthen along the spine and the back of the neck.

2. Breathe out, contract the abdominals, drop the shoulders and pull the shoulderblades down into your back as you raise the upper body away from the floor, using the muscles of the upper back, keeping the neck long and focusing your eyes forward and down. As you lift the upper body, allow the hands to lift up from the floor very slightly and reach the fingertips down towards your feet, palms facing in towards the body. At the same time bring the heels in and squeeze the inner thighs together.

3. Keeping your abdominals contracted, your shoulders dropped and your shoulderblades pulled down, breathe in and relax back down, allowing your heels to drop back out to the sides and resting your forehead on the floor, but this time facing to the other side. Repeat 5 times.

OPTION

To increase the intensity of the stretch, try this variation: breathe out as you raise up, then hold your position as you breathe in, then breathe out, contracting the abdominals, as you lower back down.

Heel Kicks

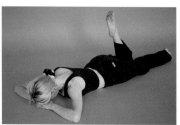

Keep lengthening along the spine and back of the neck as you kick the legs

2

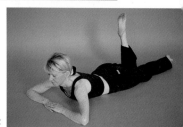

Option 2

CAUTION

- Do not attempt this exercise if you suffer from any knee or back problems.
- If you suffer from knee stiffness, try stretching the heel slowly towards the buttock, instead of kicking.

. Lie face down, with your neck lengthened and forehead resting on your hands, elbows pointing out to the sides, your legs in parallel and slightly apart. Breathe in.

> **BENEFITS**
> - Stretches the thigh muscles
> - Strengthens arms, chest muscles, hip flexors and hamstrings

2. Breathe out, contract the abdominals and kick the right heel towards the right buttock, making sure that the hips and thighs remain in contact with the floor. Release the leg slightly then kick once more.

3. Breathe in and lower the right leg, lengthening the knee away from the hip as you lower.

4. Repeat for the left leg, then repeat the entire sequence 5 to 10 times.

OPTION 1

To intensify the stretch, flex the raised foot as you kick the heel towards the buttock.

OPTION 2

For a more challenging version of this exercise, repeat the above sequence with your head lifted up away from your hands, your shoulders dropped and your upper body supported on your forearms. Lengthen along the spine and back of the neck, and focus your eyes down to your hands.

Leg Pull

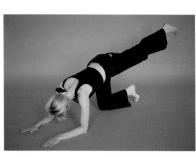

Focus your eyes straight down to help stabilise you

2

Make sure your neck is lengthened and your shoulders dropped as you work the legs

Keep the hips and shoulders level throughout this sequence – don't let your hips sink towards the floor as you raise the leg or raise your bottom higher than your shoulders

BENEFITS

- Strengthens the abdominals, the back, the shoulders and the arms
- Stretches and strengthens the legs
- Improves balance and stability

. Position yourself face down on your hands and knees with your forearms resting on the floor, your hips and shoulders level and your toes tucked under, feet slightly apart. Focus your eyes straight down to the floor, drop your shoulders away from your ears and draw your shoulderblades down into your back. Breathe in and lengthen along the spine and back of the neck.

. Breathe out, contract your abdominals and extend your left leg straight up behind you, keeping the left knee soft and the foot flexed. Keep your hips level throughout – lengthen the left leg out of the hip joint as you lift, do not let the left hip raise up too.

. Breathe in and lower the left leg, continuing to lengthen down the back of the leg and out through the heel as you do so. Repeat the lift 5 times with the left leg, then switch legs and repeat 5 times with the right.

OPTION

Once you have developed sufficient strength and stability in the abdominals and upper body, you can try this challenging variation. Repeat the exercise, this time straightening your arms and legs and raising yourself up onto your hands and feet. Check that your hands are directly below your shoulders. Keep lengthening along the back of the neck. Breathe out, contract the abdominals and raise the legs in turn, as before.

Plank

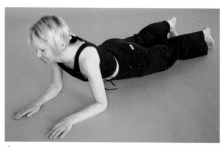

3

Keep your hips level and the spine lengthened as you raise yourself up away from the ground

As you lift up, make sure you don't raise your hips higher than your shoulders or drop them down towards the floor

---

CAUTION

Do not attempt this exercise if you suffer from any problems with your neck, back or wrists. Seek medical advice if you are in any doubt.

BENEFITS

- Strengthens the abdominals, the lower back, the upper body, the arms and the legs
- Opens out the chest and strengthens chest muscles
- Improves balance and posture
- Develops core stability
- Releases tension in the neck and shoulders

Position yourself face down with your forearms resting on the floor, hands either side of your shoulders, feet hip-width apart. Drop your shoulders and draw your shoulderblades down into your back. Lengthen along the spine and neck. Focus your eyes straight down to the floor in front of you and breathe in.

Breathe out and contract your lower abdominals as you lift up onto your knees and hands, keeping your focus downwards and your spine and neck lengthened.

Still using the outbreath, tuck your toes under and raise yourself up away from the floor, keeping your legs straight, your spine lengthened and your shoulderblades drawn down into your back. Breathe in as you lower yourself back down to the floor. Repeat 5 to 10 times.

Swan Position

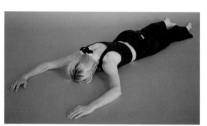

1

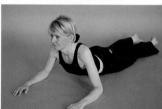

Keep the spine and neck lengthened throughout this sequence – do not curve the back as you lift

BENEFITS

- Strengthens the back and legs
- Increases strength and flexibility in the upper back, arms and shoulders
- Tones the buttocks, thighs and hips
- Improves muscle control

1. Lie face down with your forehead resting on the floor, and your legs and arms stretched away from you, slightly wider than hip- or shoulder-width apart. Your feet should be softly pointed and your elbows slightly bent.

2. Drop your shoulders down away from your ears and pull your shoulderblades down into your back. Breathe in.

3. Breathe out, contract the abdominals and, keeping your eyes focused down to the ground, lengthen up through the chest and raise the upper body slightly, keeping the forearms in contact with the floor. Breathe in and lower the body back down. Repeat 5 times.

4. Breathe out, contract the abdominals, lengthen through the chest, raising the upper body away from the floor and this time allowing the arms to raise up from the floor slightly. Breathe in and lower. Repeat 5 times.

5. Now, keeping your forehead in contact with the floor, adjust your hand position, so that your hands are palms down, slightly above your shoulders. Breathe out, contract the abdominals, and, without moving the arms or head, lengthen the legs away from you, squeezing the buttocks and allowing the legs to raise up from the floor a little. Breathe as you release the legs back down. Repeat 5 times.

Side Bend

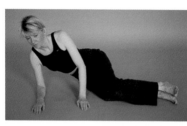

1

Do not sink your weight into your wrist and shoulder

3

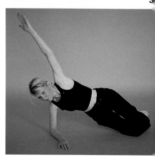

Avoid letting the hips drop to the floor or tilt forward as you lift the torso up away from the floor

As you stretch, avoid tilting the uppermost shoulder forward or arching the back

CAUTION

Do not attempt this exercise if you suffer from any wrist or shoulder problems.

BENEFITS

- Improves muscle control and balance
- Increases flexibility
- Stretches the waistline and hips

1. Sit on your right side with your knees bent, legs in parallel, knees, ankles and feet together. Place your right forearm on the floor, elbow directly below the shoulder and the hand pointing straight out. Rest your left arm on the floor in front of you. Keep your eyes focussed forwards throughout this exercise.

2. Breathe in, lengthen spine and neck and lift the ribs slightly.

3. Breathe out, contract the abdominals and raise your hips up away from the floor until the body is in a straight line, with the torso and the upper right arm forming a triangle with the floor. If this is too difficult for you to achieve at this stage, lift the hips as high as you can, keeping the movement controlled. Use the fingertips of the left hand to help you balance.

4. Breathe in, check that your shoulders are dropped and draw the shoulderblades down into the back. Keeping the pressure on the right elbow and knee, breathe out, contract the abdominals and allow the left arm to curve slowly upwards and over your head, creating a stretch along the left side of the body.

The left elbow should be soft and the hand relaxed. Only take the arm as far as you can while keeping the movement controlled and the body in alignment.

5. Breathe in as you bring the arm back down and lower the hips to the floor.

6. Repeat 5 to 10 times then change sides and repeat the sequence.

OPTION 1

If you find it too difficult to maintain your balance and lift the arm at the same time, practice the exercise just lifting and lowering the hips. As your balance gradually improves and you gain confidence, try adding the arm movement once more.

OPTION 2

Once you have developed sufficient strength and control, try the exercise with the legs extended and the left foot crossed over the right ankle and placed flat down on the floor. Raise yourself up off the floor, pressing down into the floor with your right hand and your left foot, straightening the right arm and making sure that the spine and neck are aligned.

Pillow Squeeze 2

The spine and neck should be long, with the back in the neutral position throughout

Relax your neck and make sure you do not clench your jaw

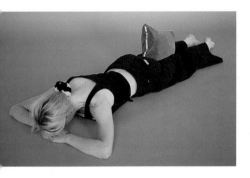

Avoid hunching the shoulders or lifting the shoulderblades – the aim of this exercise is to work the muscles in the lower body while keeping the upper body as relaxed as possible

Lengthen out of the hips and down through the legs and feet as you work the buttocks, inner thighs and abdominal core

BENEFITS

- Strengthens the muscles of the inner thighs, the abdominal muscles, the buttocks and the pelvic floor

1. Lie on your front with a cushion placed between your thighs. Position your feet so that they are pointing away from the body with the toes together and the heels dropped out to the side. Make sure that your back is straight, with your hips and shoulders parallel to each other and not tilting to one side. Check that your hips are level, with both hips in contact with the floor. Place your hands, one on top of the other, palms down, on the floor, under your forehead, elbows pointing out to the sides. Drop your shoulders away from your ears. Breathe in.

2. Breathe out, contract the abdominals (drawing them up away from the floor very slightly, but keeping the back in neutral) and squeeze the cushion together with your inner thighs, tightening the buttocks and pressing your heels in together as you. Hold for a count of 5 then breathe in and release, allowing the heels to drop out to the sides once more. Repeat the squeeze 5 times.

SITTING/KNEELING EXERCISES

Spine Stretch

Keep your shoulders down and your shoulderblades drawn down into your back

Keep the legs as straight as possible throughout this movement but do not lock the knees

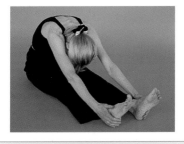

BENEFITS

- Mobilises and stretches the spine
- Releases tension in the back
- Stretches the hamstrings

TIPS

- Choose whether you do this exercise with flexed or pointed feet. The flexed-foot position will give a more intense stretch in the backs of the legs.

- If your hamstrings are very tight and you find it too uncomfortable to sit with your legs extended, then bend your knees a little (drawing your feet in towards the body), place the soles of your feet together and drop your knees out to the side.

1. Sit in an upright position with your legs slightly apart and your spine and neck lengthened. Straighten your legs, but keep your knees soft. Rest your hands on your thighs. Breathe in.

2. Breathe out, contract the abdominals, tilt the pelvis forward slightly and lengthen the back up out of the hips.

3. Still using the outbreath, drop your chin slightly towards your chest and curve forwards and down towards your thighs, rolling down through the spine one vertebra at a time and allowing the hands to slide forwards along your legs towards your feet as you stretch. Try not to collapse the ribs at the front of the body as you curve the body over – think of lifting your torso over a large inflatable beach ball.

4. Repeat the sequence 3 to 5 times.

Spine Twist

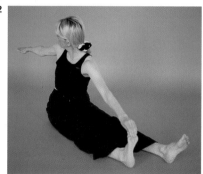

Do not collapse the upper body as you stretch forwards – lift up out of your waist and curve the body over as if you were stretching over a large beach ball

BENEFITS

- Mobilises and strengthens the upper back
- Improves flexibility
- Relieves tightness in the spine
- Gently stretches the inner thighs

CAUTION

Sit with your legs as wide apart as you can, but making sure that the position is comfortable for you – remember, the purpose of this exercise is to work the upper body, not to stretch the inner thighs.

1. Sit on the floor with your legs fairly wide apart. Drop your shoulders away from your ears and draw your shoulderblades down into your back. Breathe in, contract your abdominals, tilt your pelvis forward slightly and raise your arms to just below shoulder level, so that they are parallel to your legs. Keep the arms straight and the elbows soft.

2. Exhale and twist your upper body round to the right, so that your torso is parallel to the right leg, then lengthen your left arm forward over your right leg towards the foot, taking your right arm back behind you. Your hips should remain stationary and your legs and feet relaxed.

3. Breathe in and release to come back to centre, then breathe out and twist the upper body to the left this time, reaching the right arm towards the left foot as you take the left arm back behind you. Breathe in and return to centre once more. Repeat the sequence 5 to 10 times on each side, trying to increase the stretch each time.

Rolling Back

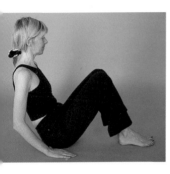

2

Keep your knees tucked in towards your chest and allow the momentum of the move, and the abdominal muscles, to bring you back to the sitting position

3

Make sure the movement is as smooth and even as possible, in time with the breathing

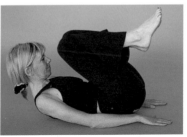

CAUTION

- If your lower back is tight or stiff, or you find this exercise too difficult, focus on the Rolling Up exercise instead, to improve your strength.
- Do not attempt this exercise if you have any neck problems or discomfort.

1. Sit on the floor with your legs bent, knees and ankles together, feet flat on the floor. Place your hands, palms down, on the floor, either side of your hips. Breathe in.

BENEFITS

- Works the abdominals
- Mobilises the lower back
- Improves muscle control

2. Breathe out, contract your abdominals, tilt your pelvis forward and slowly start to roll back, keeping your hands on the floor beside you, tucking your chin in to your chest, lengthening your neck and focusing your eyes straight ahead.

3. Continue rolling back down to the floor, allowing your feet to come away from the floor and tucking your knees into your chest.

4. Breathe in and roll back up to a sitting position, still keeping your abdominals contracted and allowing the momentum of the movement to bring you back. Press down with your hands to help you, if necessary. Repeat 5 to 10 times.

Rolling Like A Ball

Keep your knees tucked in towards your chest and allow the momentum of the move and the abdominal muscles to bring you back to the sitting position

Depending on your flexibility, you may prefer to hold the outsides of ankles instead of your thighs

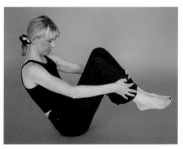

3

Make sure the movement is smooth and even as you roll backwards and forwards

CAUTION

This is challenging for some, particularly those with weak abdominals and tightness in the lower back – avoid it until you can do the Rolling Back exercise with ease. Do not attempt it if you have neck problems.

1. Sit on the floor with your legs bent, knees and ankles together, feet on the floor. Grasp the backs of the thighs with your hands. Breathe in.

> **BENEFITS**
> - Strengthens the abdominal core
> - Mobilises the spine
> - Releases tightness in the lower back

2. Breathe out, contract your abdominals, tilt your pelvis forward and slowly start to roll back, controlling the move with the abdominals and curving the lower back as you roll. Tuck your chin in to your chest slightly, lengthen along the neck and focus your eyes straight out in front of you.

3. Continue rolling through the spine, one vertebra at a time, like a ball, allowing your feet to come off the floor as you roll, keeping your knees tucked into your chest. Keep your hands in position on your ankles.

4. When you reach your furthest point (without rolling any further than onto the shoulders), breathe in and use the abdominals to roll back up to sitting – momentum will help you, but it is the abdominals that control the movement. Repeat 5 to 10 times.

OPTION

Once you have mastered this move, try starting from a balanced sitting position with your feet raised, initiating the move from your abdominals instead of pushing off from the floor with your feet.

Rocker

CAUTION

- Do not attempt this exercise until you have fully mastered Rolling Like A Ball (pp. 141–2).
- If this exercise is too challenging for you, practise Rolling Back (pp. 139–40) and Rolling Like A Ball (pp. 141–2) to improve spinal strength and flexibility.
- Avoid this exercise if you have any neck problems.

2

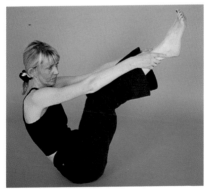

BENEFITS

- Mobilises the spine
- Builds strength in the abdominal area and legs
- Stretches the hamstrings
- Improves balance and stability

1. Sit upright with your legs in front of you, slightly apart, knees bent and feet flat on the floor. Lengthen up through the spine, drop the shoulders and draw the shoulderblades down into your back. Place your hands around your ankles and lift your legs off the floor slightly, one at a time, keeping your knees apart and bringing your toes together, into a balanced position.

2. Breathe in and lengthen up through the spine and neck, then breathe out, contract the abdominals, tilt the pelvis forward, and extend your legs, keeping the knees soft and the toes softly pointed. Extend the legs only as far as you can without losing control or balance – it is much more important for you to maintain the correct position than it is for you to straighten the legs. If it is too difficult for you to hold your ankles, then hold your calves instead.

3. Once you have extended the legs as far as you are able, breathe in, then breathe out, contract the abdominals and lower the legs back down, one at a time. Repeat 5 times, without touching the floor with your toes, if possible.

OPTION

When you have developed good balance, strength in the abdominals and flexibility in the lower back, you are ready to take this exercise further:

1. With the legs extended, exhale, contract the abdominals, tilt the pelvis forward and roll down through the spine, vertebra by vertebra, in a smooth, even movement. Keep the spine lengthened. Focus your eyes forward to help you balance.

2. Continue rolling back, taking your legs over your head – the legs should be straight, if possible with the knees soft. When you have reached your furthest point, breathe in, then breathe out and rock back to the sitting position, controlling the movement with the abdominals and allowing the momentum of the move to help you. Repeat 5 to 10 times.

Option

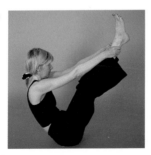

Opposite Arm & Leg Stretch

BENEFITS

- Improves strength and stability
- Improves posture and balance
- Tones the legs, buttocks and hips
- Stretches the spine

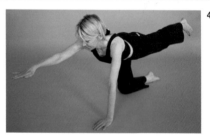

4

Make sure your hips remain stable as you extend the legs

Keep the neck lengthened throughout

Do not raise the legs or arms too high, keep them in level with the hips and shoulders – think of lengthening them out of the hip and shoulder joints, rather than lifting them

1. Position yourself on all fours, with hands beneath your shoulders and knees directly beneath your hips.

2. Drop your shoulders down away from your ears and pull your shoulderblades down into your back.

3. Breathe in and lengthen along the spine and neck, focusing your eyes straight down to the floor.

4. Breathe out, contract the abdominals and lengthen the right arm and left leg, sliding them away from you, then raising them off the ground to approximately the same level as the hips and shoulders, keeping the elbows soft as you lengthen and making sure that the arms and legs stay in line with the body.

5. Breathe in and release back down, then repeat for the other arm and leg. Repeat the sequence 5 to 10 times, using opposite arms and legs each time and alternating with each repetition.

OPTION 1

If you have difficulty balancing, try lifting the limbs one at a time (right arm, then left leg, then left arm, then right leg), until your balance improves.

OPTION 2

To increase the intensity of the movement, try holding the extended position (with one arm and one leg raised), breathe in, then breathe out, contract the abdominals and lower the arm and leg back down to the starting position.

Shoulder Stretch

Make sure you keep the abdominal contraction both as you stretch the arm through behind you and as you bring it back again

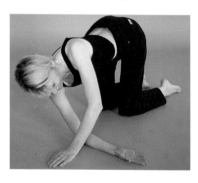

3

Keep the feet on the ground throughout this exercise, with the knees and feet in parallel and the weight evenly distributed over both knees

CAUTION

Do not attempt this exercise if you suffer from any knee complaints or have sustained any injury to the knees. Seek medical advice if you are in any doubt.

BENEFITS

- Stretches the upper back and across the shoulders
- Releases tension in the upper back
- Creates a gentle stretch in the spine

1. Kneel on the floor on all fours, with your knees directly below your hips and your hands directly beneath your shoulders. Lengthen along the spine and neck and focus the eyes down towards the floor.

2. Breathe in and transfer your weight onto your right hand. Lift your left hand and then position it so that it is placed palm upwards with the back of the hand resting on the floor.

3. Breathe out, contract the abdominals and slide the left hand through the gap under your right shoulder, taking the hand through as far as you can, following the movement of the hand with your eyes. You should feel a stretch across the upper back and shoulders. Only take the hand through as far as you can without losing your balance or losing the abdominal control. It is much more important for you to practise this exercise keeping the correct alignment than it is for you to over-reach yourself and struggle to keep control.

4. Breathe in and, maintaining the abdominal contraction, draw the arm back to the starting position. Repeat 3 to 5 times then repeat for the other side.

Side Stretch

Do not worry if you are unable to stretch very far at first, as your flexibility increases you will automatically be able to stretch the body further over towards the knee

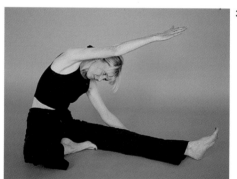

3

Keep lengthening up through the spine and along the back of the neck throughout this movement

If you find it difficult to keep the extended leg straight at first, bend the knees slightly

BENEFITS

- Stretches and tones the waist
- Stretches and strengthens the legs
- Improves flexibility
- Releases tension and tightness in the hamstrings and the lower back
- Mobilises the spine

. Sit on the floor, with your legs apart, knees soft and arms stretched out to the sides just below shoulder level. Bend your right knee and bring your right foot in to rest against the inner thigh of the left leg.

. Breathe in and lengthen up through the spine and neck.

. Breathe out, contract the abdominals and raise the right arm and curve it over your head as you lift up out of your waist and stretch the upper body up and over towards the left knee (as if you were stretching over a large beach ball).

. Hold the position and breathe in, then breathe out and increase the stretch.

. Breathe in and release the arm and bring the body back to centre. Repeat the stretch 5 times, trying to increase the stretch with each repetition, then change your leg position and repeat the entire sequence for the other side.

Tricep Dip

BENEFITS

- Strengthens and stretches the arm muscles
- Improves posture and alignment
- Develops muscle control
- Strengthens the abdominal core and the leg muscles
- Improves breath control

Keep the shoulders directly above the hips throughout

Continue to lengthen along the spine and neck as you raise and lower the body

3

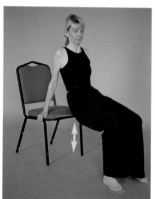

Do not lower yourself all the way to the floor – this strength-building exercise should be a slow, controlled, continuous movement, so keep the tailbone at least a few inches above the floor

CAUTION

Avoid this if you have wrist or shoulder problems.

. Position yourself about 18 inches/45cms in front of a sturdy chair, facing away from it. Place your feet hip-width apart, in parallel, toes pointing forwards.

. Grasp hold of the front corners of the seat and adjust your feet so that your ankles are directly below your knees, with your knees at right-angles, thighs parallel to the floor.

. Breathe in and lengthen along the spine and neck, drop the shoulders and draw the shoulderblades down into your back. Keep your arms straight and elbows soft. Focus your eyes straight in front of you.

. Breathe out, contract the abdominals, bend your elbows and slowly lower your tailbone to the floor, making sure your that your spine and neck remain in a line, with your hips directly below your shoulders. Lower yourself as far as you are able while keeping the abdominal contraction and maintaining control.

. When you have reached your furthest position, breathe in as you raise yourself back up to the 'sitting' position once again. Repeat 3 to 5 times.

OPTION

Try the same exercise with the knees and ankles together, squeezing the inner thighs and the buttocks as you lower and raise.

Hip Flexor Stretch

1

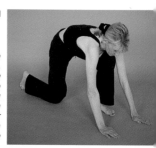

Breathe into the stretch, allowing the outbreath to take you into a deeper stretch each time

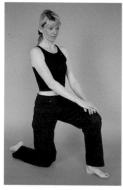

Keep the body facing forwards – avoid twisting to one side or the other as you stretch

3

BENEFITS

- Strengthens and stretches the hip flexor muscles, the hamstrings, the quadriceps and the gluteals
- Improves balance
- Releases tightness in the pelvic area

. Stand with your feet apart. Bend the knees and place your hands on the floor. Step back with the right foot, extending the leg back as far as you can, then lowering the knee to the floor, making sure that the knee and foot are in line with the right hip.

. Breathe in and bring the hands up to rest on the left knee.

. Exhale, contract the abdominals, and lengthen the body forward over the left knee, to create a stretch through the front of the left thigh. Keep the lengthening up through the spine and neck as you stretch. Breathe in and release. Repeat the stretch 5 to 10 times, breathing out as you stretch forward and breathing in as you release. Repeat for the other leg.

. To increase the stretch still further, breathe in, tuck the toes of the right foot under and raise the right knee up away from the floor. Exhale as you lengthen the body forward over the left knee increase the stretch. Inhale and release. Repeat this stretch 5 to 10 times. Repeat for the other side.

Glut Stretch

Keep the upper body, neck and shoulders as relaxed as possible throughout this stretch

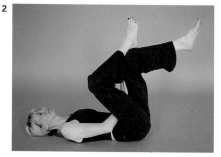

If you are unable to hold the ankle in position on the opposite knee, then take the ankle further up the leg, closer to the body

TIP
- Muscles should always be stretched out after you have finished any sequence of strengthening exercises

BENEFITS

Stretches the gluteal muscles and the lower back

Reduces tightness and stiffness in the lower back

Improves flexibility

Lie on your back with your legs bent, knees pointing to the ceiling and your arms by your sides. Breathe in and float the legs up, one at a time, towards the chest. Cross the right ankle over the left knee. Place the hands around the left thigh. Lengthen along the spine and back of your neck and focus your eyes up to the ceiling.

Breathe out, contract the abdominals, and pull your left thigh gently in towards the body, stretching the muscles in the right thigh. Hold this stretch for 5 to 10 breaths, drawing the leg closer to the chest each time you breathe out. Breathe in and release the legs back to the starting position.

Repeat on the other side.

CAUTION

If you feel any pain in your lower back, stop and release the legs a little – you may be trying to work too hard for your current level of ability. If the discomfort continues, stop and, if necessary, seek medical advice

Foot Exercises

BENEFITS
- Strengthens and mobilises the feet and ankles
- Improves circulation to the legs

TIPS
- These exercises can be done at any time and only take a few minutes – either standing or sitting whichever is most convenient.
- Keep your breathing slow and even.
- Do not roll the feet in to the centre or out to the sides.

Lifting The Arches

1. Place your feet on the floor in parallel and extend the toes.

2. Draw the toes slowly back along the floor towards you, lifting the arches.

3. Release the arches and lengthen the toes. Repeat 10 times.

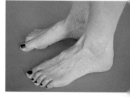

Toe Flexes

Place your feet on the floor in parallel and extend the toes.

Flex the toes up as far as you can, keeping the rest of the foot in contact with the floor.

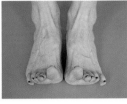

Release and extend the toes. Repeat 10 times.

Toe Teaser

Place your feet on the floor in parallel and extend the toes, spreading them as wide as you can.

Lift the big toes, leaving the other toes on the floor.

Switch and place the big toes on the floor as you lift the rest of the toes. Repeat 10 times.

Now, try lifting each toe in turn, starting with the big toe, then releasing it back to the floor and lifting the next toe, and so on. Repeat 5 to 10 times. If you cannot manage this at first, use your hands to lift each toe.

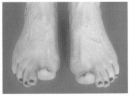

Marching Feet

1. Place your feet on the floor, ankles together, and extend the toes.

2. Raise the ball of one foot, keeping the heel on the ground.

3. Roll down through the foot, placing the ball of the foot on the ground and raising the heel.

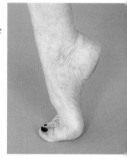

4. Repeat 5 times, then switch and repeat for the other foot.

5. Lift the toes of your right foot as you lift the heel of the left (see illustration).

6. Roll down through the feet, raising the heel of you right foot as you lift the toes of your left in a 'marching' motion.

7. Repeat 10 times.

Spinal Twist

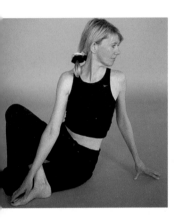

Do not take the head around any further than the shoulders as you twist and stretch

Sit upright, with your shoulders directly above your hips – do not lean back as you twist around

Avoid letting your weight sink into the floor – keep lifting up through the waist up and out of the hips

BENEFITS

- Stretches and strengthens the spine
- Releases neck, shoulder and lower-back tension
- Stretches the muscles of the hips and buttocks

1. Sit on the floor with your knees raised, feet on the floor. Tuck your right foot under your left hip and bring your left foot around, placing it next to your right thigh, with your left foot pointing forwards.

2. Start to twist your upper body around to the right slightly and place your left arm along the inside of your left calf. Breathe in.

3. Breathe out, contract the abdominals and twist around to the right with your shoulders and upper body, looking over your right shoulder and placing the fingertips of your right hand on the floor, slightly behind you, to steady you. Stay sitting upright, directing the crown of your head up to the ceiling – do not lean back. Keep your shoulders dropped and your shoulderblades drawn down into your back. Press with the left arm against the inside of the left thigh to help you twist. Hold this position for a count of 5, then breathe in and release – repeat 3 to 5 times in total, breathing out as you twist and stretch and breathing in as you release back to centre.

4. Switch positions, tucking your left foot under your right hip, placing your right foot next to your left thigh, your right arm against your right inner thigh and then placing the fingertips of your left hand on the floor to steady you as you twist and stretch around to the left, this time looking over your left shoulder. Repeat the stretch 3 to 5 times on this side.

The Cat

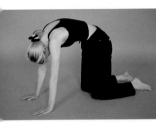

2

If your knees are uncomfortable in this pose, place a small cushion or folded towel under them

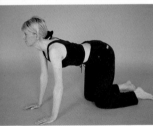

3

BENEFITS

- Relieves tension in the back and shoulders
- Improves posture
- Stretches the chest and shoulders
- Strengthens the arms

CAUTION

Beware of over-arching as you release down, as this can cause pressure in the lower back

---

1. Kneel on all fours with your knees positioned directly below your hips, and your hands directly below your shoulders, with your fingers pointing forward away from the body. The feet should rest on the ground in line with the hips and shoulders, toes pointing away from the body. Keep the arms straight and the elbows soft. Breathe in and lengthen along the spine and the back of the neck.

2. Breathe out, contract the abdominals, tuck the pelvis under, and drop your chin to your chest, lengthening through the back of the neck. As you continue to breathe out, arch the upper back towards the ceiling, like a cat, stretching the entire length of the spine. Keep the hips and shoulders level.

3. Breathe in and release back to centre and then reverse the curve very slightly, lifting the tailbone to the ceiling, and flattening out at the waist – do not drop down too far, this part of the move is a release rather than a stretch. Lift the head so that the neck is in line with the spine and lengthen out along the spine. Repeat the sequence 5 to 10 times, breathing out as you arch upwards and breathing in as you release the spine back down. Use a smooth, flowing, continuous movement, in time with the breathing.

Rest Position

BENEFITS

- Gently stretches the spine
- Releases tension in the back and neck
- Improves circulation

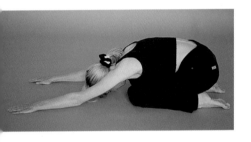

Don't worry if you are unable to sit right back on your heels at first – just reach as far as you can and let gravity to do the rest. Your hips and spine will gradually become more flexible.

CAUTION

This move should be avoided by anyone suffering from knee problems.

1. Kneel on all fours, with your knees below your hip and your hands below your shoulders, fingers pointing forward. Breathe in and lengthen along the spine and back of the neck.

2. Breathe out, contracting the abdominals, and lower your body back until you are sitting on your heels with your chest resting on the front of your thighs. Stretch your arms out in front of you in line with your shoulders.

3. Breathe in and relax your forehead down to the floor. Do not hunch the shoulders – keep them dropped down, away from the ears.

4. Hold this position for 5 to 10 breaths, allowing the spine to stretch and the body to relax a little more with every outbreath. Breathe in and come back up to centre.

OPTION

This exercise is the same as the above, except for the arm position. Experiment to find out which of the two suits you best. If you suffer from tension or stiffness in the neck and shoulders, you may find that this position is more comfortable for you. As you sit back on your heels, slide your arms back along the floor and place them close to your sides, palms facing upwards. Lengthen down through the arms, taking the hands back as far as you can, then relax the arms and shoulders as you bring the forehead down to the floor

PRACTISING PILATES

Safety

Most fitness systems these days recognise the importance of safety and have taken steps to make sure that risk of strain or injury is avoided wherever possible. However, many of the injuries that we suffer tend not to occur on the sports field or in the gym, but as we go about our daily activities – muscles can be pulled while lifting small children, bags of shopping, or even picking up a toothbrush. The Pilates technique totally retrains the body, improving posture, balance and alignment, and increasing strength, flexibility, stability and muscle control. The result of this is that we are better able to carry out our everyday activities without risk of injury.

CAUTION

If you are pregnant, if you suffer from any injury or illness, if you have recently undergone surgery, have a specific problem, or have lost or gained weight, you must seek medical advice before undertaking any new exercise regime.

Self-Awareness

The increased self-awareness that the Pilates system encourages makes us more mindful of exactly how we are using our bodies, enabling us to recognise bad habits, thus giving us the opportunity to change them. A growing self-awareness also allows us to identify any areas that require attention, so letting us strengthen and improve our weak spots.

EQUIPMENT

The Pilates technique does not necessarily require you to buy any special clothing or equipment, although various types of equipment are available should you choose to purchase them.

To practise Pilates make sure you are wearing comfortable clothing that allows you to move freely. Remember, Pilates is not a particularly strenuous type of exercise and therefore, certainly to begin with, you will need to make sure that you are wearing sufficient clothing to keep you warm as you exercise.

The only pieces of equipment that you require are:

- a folded towel, blanket or exercise mat to place on the floor to protect you – even if you are exercising on a carpeted area, it is best to give yourself a little extra padding on which to exercise;

- a scarf or stretchy rubber exercise band;

THE BENEFITS OF PILATES

- Improves mind/body awareness
- Develops the body's core abdominal strength
- Increases strength and improves balance
- Lengthens and stretches the muscles to give you a leaner body without building bulk
- Reduces stress levels and fatigue
- Improves stability, flexibility and joint mobility
- Reduces incidences of strain and injury
- Boosts the immune system
- Gives an increased sense of well-being
- Improves circulation and muscle tone
- Enhances muscle control without causing tension
- Improves the functioning of the respiratory and lymphatic systems
- Relieves headaches and can help eliminate the cause of stress-, tension-, or posture-related headaches
- Improves bone density
- Relieves pain, stiffness and tension
- Exercises the muscles without causing pain or risking muscle tears or strains or jarred joints
- Teaches you to enjoy the movements as you stretch
- Is suitable for anyone, regardless of age or level of fitness
- The fundamental principles of the Pilates method can be applied to any movement or activity

- a flat cushion, or small folded towel to place under your head, if necessary.

Specialist equipment and clothing are available from most Pilates organisations. Check on their websites or telephone them for further details. Some useful address and websites are given in the back of this book (pp. 190–2).

TIP

Remember, exercise can only have a lasting effect if you make it an ongoing part of your weekly routine. Only by committing to a programme of regular exercise, a healthy diet, and sufficient sleep, can you effect permanent positive changes to your level of fitness, your body shape and your general well-being.

PILATES FOR A HEALTHY BODY

'The best exercise is the one you do.'

Edgar Cayce

Plan your exercise routine to suit your lifestyle and be realistic about what you will actually be able to achieve. Is it easier and more efficient for you to exercise for a few minutes each day, rather than one long weekly session? Or would a longer session suit you better?

Organise a programme of exercise for yourself that you will easily be able to fulfil each week: there is no point in setting yourself impossible goals that only leave you feeling frustrated when you are unable to meet them, or that push you too hard and leave you feeling exhausted and burnt out.

The most important factor is your willingness to commit to a regular exercise programme (regardless of how much or little time you have available), and to making positive changes in your daily life. Only with consistent practice will you truly begin to notice lasting changes to your body shape, your fitness levels, your health and your feeling of well-being. Remember, though, the more you exercise the quicker you will see the results and the more benefit you will feel.

For Pilates to effect real and lasting changes you need to dedicate a total time of at least an hour each week to the exercise.

Best Time To Exercise

Choose a time to exercise when you will not be continually interrupted, and unplug the telephone. You might even like to put on some relaxing background music. If you are someone who finds it hard to prioritise taking time to do things for yourself and constantly find yourself intending to exercise, but always being pulled away to do something else, you might even consider booking an 'appointment' with yourself in advance for a specific time and day, which you do not allow yourself to cancel or change.

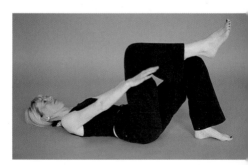

Noticing The Effects

Some people notice immediate changes with Pilates, but it usually takes around 6 to 10 sessions for most people start to notice an overall improvement in their posture, body shape, stamina, strength and flexibility.

DO NOT EXERCISE IF

- you are feeling unwell, exhausted or feverish

- you suffer from any complaint, are recovering from illness or injury, are pregnant, have recently lost or gained weight, or are on a course of treatment and have not yet sought medical advice

Planning Your Exercise Routine

In principle, the ideal time to exercise is at the end of the day, when your muscles are warmed up. But the best time to choose is the one that appeals to you most and fits best with your schedule – maybe the start of the day is the optimum time for you to exercise, preparing you for the day ahead; or perhaps you favour a relaxing wind-down in the evening, to help you let go of the stresses and strains of a hectic day.

If you choose to exercise first thing in the morning, start by rolling down against a wall (p. 36) a few times, to help mobilise your spine and gently wake up the whole body.

If you exercise in the evening, it is a good idea to begin your sessions by lying on your back, legs bent, feet flat on the floor, knees pointing up to the ceiling and concentrate on your breathing for a few minutes, to give your mind a chance to clear and your body the opportunity to relax and let go of any tensions that it has accumulated throughout the day.

As you progress and develop your strength and ability and move on to more challenging exercises, don't give up the 'easier' versions of exercises entirely. You will find it extremely useful to include these earlier moves using them as warm-ups for the harder variations, or as an opportunity to focus on improving aspects of your technique such as precision and muscle control or, by adding further repetitions, developing your stamina.

CAUTION

Always pay attention to your body as you work. Listen to any messages it may be communicating to you – if you are feeling discomfort, it is probably for a reason. Don't ever simply battle through aches and pains, always either adjust what you are doing, until you are able to practise the move in comfort and control, or, if necessary, stop the exercise you are doing entirely.

SUGGESTED ROUTINES

Short Daily Routines

If you choose to do short daily routines, once you have warmed up each day, you will not have much time to work intensively with many of the exercises. But it is better to choose fewer moves and work in a focused, controlled manner than to rush through a large number of moves and risk practising them incorrectly. Vary your daily programme so that, within the course of a week, you have included some exercises for all the different areas of the body. Here are seven suggestions to get you started; page numbers follow in italics.

SHORT DAILY ROUTINE 1

Breathing *35*	Neck pull *66*
Rolling down the wall *36*	One-leg circles *79*
Arm swings *38*	Squeezing the pillow *114*
Shoulder hunches *40*	Horizontal star *116*
Alternate hip openings *41*	Rolling back *139*
Arm raises *48*	Arm & leg stretch *146*
Waist twist *50*	Cat *163*
Push up *54*	Rest position *165*
Hundred *63*	

SHORT DAILY ROUTINE 2

Breathing *35*

Rolling down the wall *36*

Standing balance *37*

Arm raises into arm circles *39*

Alternate hip openings *41*

Hip folds *42*

Egyptian arm circles *44*

Spine curls *56*

Hundred *63*

Neck stretch *68*

Single-leg stretch *70*

Double-leg stretch *74*

Shoulder lifts *81*

Arm openings *83*

Arm circles *00*

Chest opener *52*

Spine stretch *135*

Shoulder stretch *148*

Rest position *165*

SHORT DAILY ROUTINE 3

Breathing *26*

Rolling down the wall *36*

Arm swings *38*

Alternate hip openings *41*

Hip folds *42*

Egyptian arm circles *44*

Arm raises *48*

Arm lifts *00*

Push up *54*

Hip rolls *60*

Hundred *63*

Windmill *86*

Leg lifts *100*

Double leg lifts (side) *106*

Swan position *128*

Pillow squeeze 2 *133*

Spinal twist *161*

Rest position *165*

SHORT DAILY ROUTINE 4

Breathing 35
Standing balance 37
Arm raises into arm circles 39
Shoulder hunches 40
Egyptian arm circles 44
Arm raises 48
Hip rolls 60
Hundred 63
Neck pull 66
Neck stretch 68
Single-leg stretch 70

Double-leg stretch 74
Hamstring stretch 77
Inner thigh stretch 108
Horizontal star 116
Spine stretch 135
Spine twist 137
Rolling like a ball 141
Hip flexor stretch 154
Glut stretch 156
Foot exercises 158

SHORT DAILY ROUTINE 5

Breathing 35
Rolling down the wall 36
Arm swings 38
Shoulder hunches 40
Alternate hip openings 41
Hip folds 42
Hip rolls 60
Hundred 63
Push up 54
Neck pull 66
Double-leg stretch 74
Corkscrew 88

Jack knife 90
Rolling up 98
Ankle circles 112
Squeezing the pillow 114
One-leg heel kicks 122
Shoulder press 118
Dart 120
Leg pull 124
Arm and leg stretch 146
Cat 163
Rest position 165

SHORT DAILY ROUTINE 6

Breathing 26
Rolling down the wall 36
Arm raises into arm circles 39
Shoulder hunches 40
Alternate hip openings 41
Push up 54
Spine curls 56
Hip rolls 60
Hundred 63
Single-leg stretch 70
One-leg circles 79

Teaser 93
Scissors 96
Rolling over 110
Squeezing the pillow 114
Shoulder press 118
Plank 126
Side bend 130
Tricep dip 152
Arm and leg stretch 146
Shoulder stretch 148
Hip flexor stretch 154

SHORT DAILY ROUTINE 7

Breathing 35
Standing balance 37
Arm swings 38
Alternate hip openings 41
Hip folds 42
Egyptian arm circles 44
Rolling down 46
Arm raises 48
Push up 54
Spine curls 56
Hundred 63

Neck pull 66
Neck stretch 68
Single-leg stretch 70
Arm openings 83
Leg lifts 100
One-leg circles 79
Shoulder press 118
Dart 120
Rocker 143
Side stretch 150
Rest position 165

2/3 Times Weekly Routines

If you prefer to set aside longer amounts of time to devote to your exercise programme, here are a few suggestions for some longer routines. Again, make sure that you vary your sessions each time, to include some exercises for all the different areas of the body.

2/3 TIMES WEEKLY ROUTINE 1

Breathing *35*	Shoulder lifts *81*
Rolling down the wall *36*	Arm openings *83*
Standing balance *37*	Corkscrew *88*
Arm swings *38*	Teaser *93*
Shoulder hunches *40*	Rolling up *98*
Alternate hip openings *41*	Leg lifts *100*
Arms lifts *00*	Ankle circles *112*
Waist twist *50*	Squeezing the pillow *114*
Chest opener *52*	Horizontal star *116*
Push up *54*	Shoulder press *118*
Spine curls *56*	Dart *120*
Hip rolls *60*	Swan position *128*
Hundred *63*	Spine stretch *135*
Neck pull *66*	Spine twist *137*
Neck stretch *68*	Rolling back *139*
Single-leg stretch *70*	Cat *163*
Double-leg stretch *74*	Rest position *165*

2/3 TIMES WEEKLY ROUTINE 2

Breathing *35*

Arm swings *38*

Arm raises into arm circles *39*

Shoulder hunches *40*

Alternate hip openings *41*

Hip folds *42*

Egyptian arm circles *44*

Rolling down *46*

Spine curls *56*

Arm circles (standing) *58*

Hip rolls *60*

Hundred *63*

Neck pull *66*

Neck stretch *68*

One-leg circles *79*

Shoulder lifts *81*

Windmill *86*

Jack knife *90*

Teaser *93*

Rolling up *98*

Double leg lifts (side) *106*

Rolling over *110*

Rolling like a ball *141*

Rocker *143*

Dart *120*

One-leg heel kicks *122*

Leg pull *124*

Plank *126*

Pillow squeeze 2 *133*

Arm and leg stretch *146*

Shoulder stretch *148*

Tricep dip *152*

Cat *163*

Rest position *165*

2/3 TIMES WEEKLY ROUTINE 3

Breathing *35*

Arm raises into arm circles *39*

Shoulder hunches *40*

Alternate hip openings *41*

Hip folds *42*

Egyptian arm circles *44*

Rolling down *46*

Waist twist *50*

Spine curls *56*

Hip rolls *60*

Hamstring stretch *77*

Single-leg stretch *70*

Double-leg stretch *74*

One-leg circles *79*

Shoulder lifts *81*

Hundred *63*

Hamstring stretch *77*

Jack knife *90*

Scissors *96*

Inner thigh stretch *108*

Squeezing the pillow *114*

Horizontal star *116*

Shoulder press *118*

Dart *120*

Side bend *130*

Spine stretch *135*

Rolling back *139*

Rolling like a ball *141*

Side stretch *150*

Hip flexor stretch *154*

Glut stretch *156*

Foot exercises *158*

Spinal twist *161*

Rest position *165*

Weekly Routines

The following routines are a few suggestions for those people who wish to work at one longer weekly session per week, or for those who have chosen to do two longer sessions per week than the ones given above.

WEEKLY ROUTINE 1

Breathing 26	Rolling over 110
Rolling down the wall 36	Ankle circles 112
Standing balance 37	Horizontal star 116
Arm swings 38	Shoulder press 118
Arm raises into arm circles 39	Dart 120
Shoulder hunches 40	One-leg heel kicks 122
Alternate hip openings 41	Leg pull 124
Hip folds 42	Plank 126
Egyptian arm circles 44	Swan position 128
Arm raises 48	Side bend 130
Waist twist 50	Spine stretch 135
Push up 54	Spine twist 137
Spine curls 56	Rolling back 139
Hip rolls 60	Rocker 143
Hundred 63	Side stretch 150
Neck pull 66	Hip flexor stretch 154
Single-leg stretch 70	Foot exercises 158
Double-leg stretch 74	Spinal twist 161
Arm openings 83	Cat 163
Jack knife 90	Rest position 165

WEEKLY ROUTINE 1 (CONT'D)

WEEKLY ROUTINE 2

FURTHER INFORMATION

Further Reading

- **10 Step Pilates**: Reshape Your Body and Transform Your Life, Lesley Ackland, Thomas Paton, Malu Halasa, Thorsons, 2001

- **15 Minute Pilates**: Body Maintenance to Make You Longer, Leaner and Stronger, Lesley Ackland, Eva Gizowska, HarperCollins, 2001

- **A Pilates' Primer**: The Millennium Edition, Joseph H. Pilates, William J. Miller, Bodymind Publishing, 2000

- **Abdominal Training**, Christopher M. Norris, Lyons Press, 2002

- **Back Stability**, Christopher M. Norris, Human Kinetics Europe, 2000

- **Body Control: the Pilates Way**, Lynne Robinson, Pan, 1998

- **The Body Control Pilates Back Book**, Lynne Robinson, Paul Massey, Pan, 2002

- **Complete Guide to the Pilates Method,** Allan Menezes, Peter Green, Hunter House, 2000

Complete Idiot's Guide to the Pilates Method, Karon Karter, Colleen Glen, Pearson Education, 2000

Complete Writings of Joseph H. Pilates: Return to Life through Contrology and Your Health – the Authorized Edition, Joseph H. Pilates, John Miller, Sean P. Gallagher (ed.), BainBridgeBooks, 2000

Emily Kelly's Commonsense Pilates, Emily Kelly, Anness Publishing, 2000

Every Body is Beautiful, Ron Fletcher, Lippencott, 1978

Everything Pilates, Amy Taylor Taylor Alpers, Lorna Gentry, Rachel Taylor Segel, Adams Media Corporation, 2002

How to Improve Your Posture, Fran Lehen, Cornerstone Library, 1982

In-Flight Fitness, Dreas Reyneke and Helen Varley, Vermillion, 2001

Intelligent Exercise with Pilates & Yoga, Lynne Robinson and Howard Napper, Macmillan 2002

Jennifer Kries' Pilates Plus Method: The Unique Combination of Yoga, Dance and Pilates, Jennifer Kries, Warner Books, 2002

Joseph H. Pilates Archive Collection: Photographs, Writings and Designs, Sean P. Gallagher (ed.), Romana Kryzanowska (ed.), BainBridge Books, 2000

- **The Joseph H. Pilates Method at Home**: A Balance Shape, Strength, and Fitness Program, Eleanor McKenzie, Trevor Blount, Ulysses Press, 2000

- **Little Pilates Book**, Erika Dillman, Warner Books, 2001

- **The Mind Body Workout: Pilates and the Alexander Technique**, Lynne Robinson, Helge Fisher, Pan, 1998

- **The Official Body Control Fitness Manual**, Lynne Robinson, Gordon Thompson, MacMillan, 2002

- **Perfect Body the Pilates Way**, Lynne Robinson, Caroline Brien, MacMillan, 2002

- **The Pilates Back Book**: Heal Neck, Back, and Shoulder Pain with Easy Pilates Stretches, Tia Stanmore, Rockport, 2002

- **The Pilates Body**, Brooke Siler, Michael Joseph, 2000

- **Pilates Body Power**, Lesley Ackland, Thorsons, 2000

- **Pilates for a Fabulous Body**, Lesley Ackland, Thorsons, 2002

- **Pilates for Beginners**, Kellina Stewart, HarperInformation, 2001

- **Pilates for Beginners**, Roger Brignall, Sterling, 2000

- **Pilates for Dummies,** Ellie Herman, Wiley, John & Sons, 2002

Pilates for Every Body, Denise Austin, Rodale Press, 2002

The Pilates Pregnancy, Mari Winsor with Mark Laska, Vermillion, 2002

Pilates for Pregnancy, Anna Selby, HarperCollins, 2002

Pilates for Pregnancy, Michael King and Yolande Green, Ulysses, 2002

Pilates Gym, Lynne Robinson and Gerry Convy, Pan, 2001

The Pilates Method of Physical and Mental Conditioning, Philip Friedman and Gail Eisen, Warner Books, 1980

Pilates on the Ball: The World's Most Popular Workout Using the Exercise Ball, Colleen Craig, Healing Art Press, 2001

Pilates Personal Trainer: Getting Started with Stretching, Michael King, Ulysses Press, 2003

The Pilates Powerhouse, Mari Winsor and Mark Laska, Vermillion, 2001

Pilates' Return to Life through Contrology, Joseph H. Pilates, William J. Miller, Judd Robbins (ed.), Bodymind Publishing, 1998

- **Pilates Workbook**: Illustrated Step-by-Step Guide to Matwork Techniques, Michael King, Ulysses Press, 2001

- **Pilates**, Cathy Meeus, Sally Searle, DK Publishing, 2001

- **Pilates**, Patricia Lamond, Globe Pequot Press, 20

- **Pilates**: Realize Your Potential and Discover Grac Power and Supple Movement with Pilates, Suzan: Scott (intro), Sterling, 2002

- **Pilates**: The Complete Body System, Michael King Mitchell Beazley, 2003

- **The Pilates Workout Journal**: An Exercise Diary and Conditioning Guide, Mari Winsor with Mark Laska, Perseus, 2001

- **Pure Pilates**, Michael King, Mitchell Beazley, 2001

- **Ultimate Pilates**, Dreas Reyneke, Vermillion, 2002

- **Your Health**: A Corrective System of Exercising tha Revolutionizes the Entire Field of Physical Education, Joseph Hubertus Pilates, Judd Robbins (ed.), Lin Van Huit-Robbins (intro), Present Dynamics, 1998

Exercise Videos/DVDs

Introduction to Pilates –The Power Within, IMC Vision Ltd, 2001

Motoner Workout Volume 1, Michael King, Pilates Institute

Pilates Express, Lynne Robinson & Pat Cash, Rank Videos

Pilates Intermediate Matwork – Volume 1, Pilates Institute

Pilates Powerhouse, Body Control 5 with Lynne Robinson, Telstar Video Entertainment, 2001

Pilates, Micah Bo, International Licensing and Copyright Ltd, 2001

Pilates: The Perfect Body & Pilates Express, Telstar Video Entertainment, 2001

Pilates-Inspired Matwork – Volumes 1–3, Terra Entertainment, 2002

Super Sculpt, Michael King

Tripower, Michael King

Yogalates, Momentum Pictures Home Entertainment, 2001

Useful Addresses

UK

The Body Control Pilates Association, PO Box 290
London WC2H 9TB
www.bodycontrol.co.uk

The Pilates Foundation UK Ltd, PO Box 36052,
London SW16 1XQ
Tel. 07071 781559
www.pilatesfoundation.com

The Alan Herdman Studio, 17 Homer Row, London
Tel. 020 7723 9953

Body Maintenance Studio, 2nd Floor, Pineapple,
7 Langley Street, London WC2H 9JA

The Pilates Institute, Wimborne House,
151–155 New North Road, London N1 6TA
www.pilates-institute.co.uk

USA

re:Ab Studio, 33 Bleecker Street, Suite 2C, New York
NY 10012
Tel. (212) 420 9111
www.reabnyc.com

Tribeca Bodyworks, 177 Duane Street, New York,
NY 10003

el. (212) 625 0777
www.tribecabodyworks.com

imate Body Control, 30 East 60th Street #606,
w York, NY 10022
w.pilates-ny.com

es Studio of Los Angeles, 8704 Santa Monica Bvd,
e 300, West Hollywood, California
(310) 659 1077
w.pilatestherapy.com

NADA

etti Studio, 1115 Sherbrooke Street West,
ntreal, Quebec
(514) 285 4884
www.pilates-montreal.com

Websites

www.allaboutpilates.com

ww.backpain.org

ww.bodymind.net

ww.bodyzone.com

ww.classicalpilates.net

ww.clinicalpilates.com/nz.htm

ww.excelpilates.com

ww.gothampilates.com

www.nzsites.com/pilates
www.peakpilates.com
www.physicalcompany.co.uk
www.physioworks.co.uk
www.pilates.ca
www.pilates.co.uk
www.pilates.com
www.pilates.net
www.pilatesbodyworksintl.com
www.pilatesdirect.com
www.pilates-marybowen.com
www.pilatesontheball.com
www.pilates-studio.com
www.powerpilates.com
www.re-balance-studio.nl
www.sagefitness.com
www.sissel-online.com
www.stottpilates.com
www.themethod.com
www.themethodpilates.com
www.thepilatescenter.com
www.thethirdspace.com
www.turningpointstudios.com
www.winsorpilates.com